MRCGP
MULTIPLE CHOICE
REVISION BOOK

Second Edition

edited by

Peter Ellis MA MMed Ed MRCGP
Medical and Educational Advisor
London

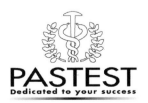

PASTEST
Dedicated to your success

© 2004 PASTEST Ltd
Egerton Court
Parkgate Estate
Knutsford
Cheshire
WA16 8DX

Telephone: 01565 752000

First published 2002
Second edition 2004

ISBN: 1 904627 32 3

A catalogue record for this book is available from the British Library.

The information contained within this book was obtained by the authors from
reliable sources. However, while every effort has been made to ensure its
accuracy, no responsibility for loss, damage or injury occasioned to any person
acting or refraining from action as a result of information contained herein can
be accepted by the publishers or authors.

PasTest Revision Books and Intensive Courses
PasTest has been established in the field of postgraduate medical education since
1972, providing revision books and intensive study courses for doctors preparing
for their professional examinations.

Books and courses are available for the following specialties:
MRCGP, MRCP Parts 1 and 2, MRCPCH Parts 1 and 2, MRCPsych, MRCS,
MRCOG Parts 1 and 2, DRCOG, DCH, FRCA, PLAB Parts 1 and 2

Typeset by Carnegie Book Production, Lancaster
Printed and bound in Europe by The Alden Group

CONTENTS

Contributors   iv

Introduction   v

MRCGP membership examination   vi

Content of the multiple choice paper   vii

Exam preparation and technique   viii

Acknowledgements   xi

MEDICINE   1

    Cardiovascular   3
    Dermatology/ENT/Ophthalmology   12
    Endocrine/Metabolic   38
    Gastroenterology/Nutrition   56
    Infectious diseases/Haematology/
      Immunology/Allergies/Genetics   65
    Paediatrics   74
    Pharmaco-therapeutics   81
    Psychiatry/Neurology   94
    Reproductive/Renal   121
    Respiratory medicine   138

ADMINISTRATION AND MANAGEMENT   159

RESEARCH, EPIDEMIOLOGY AND STATISTICS   177

MEDICINE ANSWERS   217

ADMINISTRATION AND MANAGEMENT ANSWERS   313

RESEARCH, EPIDEMIOLOGY AND STATISTICS ANSWERS   325

Index   345

CONTRIBUTORS

ROB DANIELS MA MRCGP

General Practitioner
Townsend House Medical Centre
Seaton
Devon

FIRST EDITION

ANWAR A KHAN BSc MBBS DRCOG DCH (Lond) DCCH (Edin) FRCGP

GP Trainer and course organiser
Loughton Health Centre
Loughton
Essex

and

Examiner
Royal College of General Practitioners

MAHENDRA MASHRU MSc MBBChir MRCS FRCGP

General Practitioner
Ruislip

Middlesex

and

Honorary Senior Lecturer
Imperial College School of Medicine
London

INTRODUCTION

This revision book has been written to help candidates with their preparations for the machine-marked paper of the MRCGP examination. There are questions in various formats: Extended Matching Questions, Multiple Best Answer and Single Best answer and Summary Completion Questions. All the questions are arranged by subject in sections which correspond with the headings published by the Royal College of General Practitioners in the information about the MRCGP examination. Candidates indicated to us that they would like a book of questions sorted by subject, as they find such an arrangement helpful when revising for this examination.

We have updated the material in this book and included summary completion questions and illustrated questions.

We are always happy to receive comments about our material, and we would certainly like to know if this current book has indeed been of help to you.

Good luck with the MRCGP exam!

Peter Ellis
October 2004

MRCGP MEMBERSHIP EXAMINATION

The membership examination of the Royal College of General Practitioners is constantly changing, and in the past it contained Multiple Choice Question papers, Modified Essay Question papers, Traditional Essay Questions and Practice Topic Questions.

The MRCGP examination is now a modular examination consisting of four modules:

1   Written Paper – the examiner-marked paper.
2   Multiple Choice Paper – the machine-marked paper.
3   Assessment of consulting skills.
4   Oral examination.

To be successful in the MRCGP examination candidates must pass all four modules. There is a credit accumulation system and the modules can be taken together or at different sessions and can be taken in any order. This book is written for the machine-marked written paper, Paper 2, which is available twice a year.

The machine-marked paper is designed to test knowledge and application of that knowledge by candidates. The paper contains Extended Matching Questions (EMQs), Single Best Answer Questions (SBAs), Multiple Best Answer Questions (MBAs) and Summary Completion Questions (SCQs). All answers are recorded by candidates on sheets that can be machine-marked. The Royal College states that the number of items in each format is variable, and the maximum number of items in the paper will be 250. For the most up-to-date information, see the Royal College website at www.rcgp.org.uk.

There is no negative marking for any of the question types in the machine-marked written module. There is therefore no point in leaving a question blank. It pays to guess! Questions are machine scored on a basis of +1 mark for a correct answer and 0 for a wrong or missed response.

CONTENT OF THE MULTIPLE CHOICE PAPER

Medicine

- Cardiovascular
- Dermatology/ENT/Ophthalmology
- Endocrinology/Metabolic
- Gastroenterology/Nutrition
- Infectious diseases/Haematology/Immunology/Allergies/ Genetics
- Paediatrics
- Pharmaco-therapeutics
- Psychiatry/Neurology
- Reproductive/Renal
- Respiratory

Administration and Management, including

- Regulatory framework of the NHS
- Legal aspects
- Business aspects
- Certification, benefits and allowances
- Professional regulation

Research, Epidemiology and Statistics, including

- Assessing the quality of care
- Principles of audit
- Understanding and application of the terms used in inferential statistics and evidence-based medicine
- Knowledge of statistics and research methodology, sufficient for the critical appraisal of published papers

EXAM PREPARATION AND TECHNIQUE

In trying to pass any examination it helps to plan an effective revision programme that concentrates on the elements that are being examined and not the areas which the exam cannot or does not test. There are certain basic principles which are relevant to each part of the MRCGP exam.

1   Read relevant literature.

> Remember that this is an examination of British general practice. You will gain far more from reading a book about the consultation than from reading about ENT or ophthalmology, etc in a textbook.

2   Ask yourself WHY?

> The exam asks you to appraise critically what you are doing. After every consultation ask yourself about the outcome. Did you feel happy about it, do you think the patient was satisfied with your management? If not, why not, and how could you have managed the situation better? After every article you read, ask yourself why the article was written, whether it was relevant, what the main points were that the author was trying to get across, and whether there were better ways of achieving the same result. Be critical in a constructive way about your work and your reading.

3   Form an alliance with other candidates.

> By meeting on a regular basis you can stimulate one another to be more critical. You can also divide the onerous task of ploughing through journals between the group and become much more knowledgeable very quickly. Finally, by talking to colleagues you will retain more factual knowledge and also be able to clarify your ideas and opinions more clearly.

There are also specific techniques that will help you to prepare for the machine-marked paper. It is often thought that you cannot improve your score in machine-marked examinations by repeatedly doing tests. We do not think that this is true. Candidates who do not improve their scores are using practice papers in the wrong way. What normally happens is that a candidate will spend a lot of time reading textbooks and then do a practice examination. It is far better to do an examination first, and then spend a lot of time reading around the answers and extending your knowledge in this way. Even with good teaching notes you still need to read around the topic. There are only a limited number of areas relevant to general practice on which machine-marked questions can be set and by doing a number of practice examinations in this way you can substantially increase your knowledge base and thus increase your overall score.

ON EXAMINATION DAY

By the time the day of the examination arrives you will certainly have invested a good deal of money, and probably a lot of time and effort, in the exam. It is important that you do not blow it all on the day by making silly mistakes.

Again, there are certain basic rules for approaching each part of the MRCGP.

1   Do not be tired.

> This may sound simple but if you have nights on call in the three to four days before the examination, then swap them. Try to keep your workload to a minimum. If you arrive tired you will not cope well with several hours of written work.

2   Arrive in time.

> Every year, for both the written and oral examinations, candidates underestimate the time it will take them to get to the examination venue. They arrive distressed and anxious and under these circumstances can never do themselves justice.

3   Key into the task.

> By arriving in plenty of time, you have the chance to prepare mentally for the examination. Reading a current journal quietly just before going into the exam will start your brain thinking about general practice and current issues. When you sit down to start working on the papers you will already be in the right frame of mind and this will save you valuable time.

4   Read the instructions.

> No matter how well you think you know the rules, always read the instructions at the beginning. There should be no changes from previous years but just in case there are, this is time well spent.

The majority of candidates will not be short of time in the machine-marked paper, but there are a number of special techniques which should help.

1   Read the whole paper before you answer anything. This allows a lot of subconscious recall to happen before you start to mark your answers.

2   Read every word in the stem and in each item. It is very easy to make simple mistakes by thinking that you read something that was not actually there.

3   Mark the answer sheet carefully. Do not get the answer responses out of sequence. If you do have to alter a response rub it out well and mark the new response clearly. The answer sheets are marked by machine and an inadequately rubbed out answer could be interpreted as your true response.

4   Answer every item. Remember there is NO negative marking and thus marks may be gained by guessing.

Finally, enjoy your studying using this book, and good luck with the examination!

ACKNOWLEDGEMENTS

PasTest would like to thank the BMJ Publishing Group for their kind permission to reproduce extracts from the following articles:

Logroscino et al, 'Prospective study of type 2 diabetes and cognitive decline in women aged 70-81 years,' *British Medical Journal* 2004; 328:548–51

Eaton et al, 'Coeliac disease and schizophrenia: population based case control study with linkage of Danish national registers,' *British Medical Journal* 2004; 328:438–9

Hotpf et al, 'Gulf War illness – better, worse or just the same? A cohort study,' *British Medical Journal* 2003; 327: 1370

De Jogn van den Berg et al, 'Influence of the third generation pill controversy on prescriptions for oral contraceptives among first time users: population based study,' *British Medical Journal* 2003; 326: 254

Goodacre et al, 'Randomised controlled trial and economic evaluation of a chest pain observation unit compared with routine care,' *British Medical Journal* 2004; 328:254–7

Mamdani et al, 'Observational study of upper gastrointestinal haemorrhage in elderly patients given selective cyclo-oxygenase-2 inhibitors or conventional non-steroidal anti-inflammatory drugs,' *British Medical Journal* 2002; 325: 624–7.

PasTest would also like to thank the British Journal of General Practice for their kind permission to reproduce extracts from the following articles:

Van de Laar et al, 'Fat intake in patients newly diagnosed with type 2 diabetes: a 4-year follow-up study in general practice.' *British Journal of General Practice* 2004; 54:177-82

Stratelis et al, 'Early detection of COPD in primary care: screening by invitation of smokers aged 40 - 55 years,' *British Journal of General Practice* 2004; 54: 201-6

Johnson and Helman, 'Remedy or cure? Lay beliefs about over-the-counter medicines for coughs and colds.' *British Journal of General Practice* 2004; 54: 98–102

Dey et al, 'Implementation of RCG guidelines for acute low back pain: a cluster randomised controlled trial,' *British Journal of General Practice* 2004; 54: 33–7

MEDICINE QUESTIONS

CARDIOVASCULAR

EXTENDED MATCHING QUESTIONS

THEME: PULSES

A Absent

B Bisferiens

C Collapsing

D Plateau

E Pulsus alternans

F Pulsus paradoxus

For each of the descriptions, select the most likely type of pulse. Each option may be used once, more than once, or not at all.

1 Found in aortic stenosis. ☐

2 Found in left ventricular failure. ☐

3 Found in aortic regurgitation. ☐

4 Found with mixed aortic stenosis and incompetence. ☐

5 Usually noted when taking blood pressure – doubling in rate noted as mercury level falls. ☐

6 Found with severe chronic obstructive pulmonary disease. ☐

7 Pulse volume decreases markedly with inspiration. ☐

8 This is low amplitude with slow rise and fall. ☐

THEME: ECG FINDINGS

A Absent P waves with ragged baseline

B Inverted T wave

C Large R waves in V1–V2

D Large S waves in V1–V2

E Long QT interval

F Peaked T wave

G Prolonged PR interval

H Short PR interval

I Short QT interval

For each of the descriptions, select the most likely ECG finding. Each option may be used once, more than once, or not at all.

9 Wolff–Parkinson–White syndrome. ☐

10 Atrial fibrillation. ☐

11 Hyperkalaemia. ☐

12 Right ventricular hypertrophy. ☐

13 Hypercalcaemia. ☐

14 First-degree heart block. ☐

15 Ischaemia or bundle branch block. ☐

16 Hypocalcaemia. ☐

17 Left ventricular hypertrophy. ☐

MULTIPLE BEST ANSWER QUESTIONS

1   A Mediterranean diet combines which TWO of the following?

☐ **A**   Replaces poultry with red meat

☐ **B**   Increases fish, fruit and vegetables

☐ **C**   Reduces coronary artery disease more than just a low-fat diet

2   Adults who exercise regularly have which FOUR of the following?

☐ **A**   Lower blood pressure

☐ **B**   Increased risk of cancer of the colon

☐ **C**   Less likelihood of depression

☐ **D**   Lower incidence of diabetes

☐ **E**   Improved co-ordination

3   Select THREE statements concerning events following myocardial infarction

☐ **A**   50% of deaths occur within two hours of onset of symptoms

☐ **B**   Ventricular fibrillation is most likely to occur at 48–72 hours

☐ **C**   The ECG can remain normal for several hours

☐ **D**   The ECG can remain normal for several days

☐ **E**   Thrombolytic therapy is contraindicated until chest pain has resolved

4   Which TWO of the following statements about angina pectoris are correct?

☐   **A**   May occur with normal coronary arteries

☐   **B**   Is associated with abnormal resting ECG between attacks in about 90% of cases

☐   **C**   Is typically worse later in the day

☐   **D**   ST segment elevation on ECG is usual during an attack

☐   **E**   May be aggravated by lying down

5   Select THREE of the following statements concerning deep venous thrombosis

☐   **A**   Is not common in patients over the age of 40

☐   **B**   Has been linked to long-haul flights

☐   **C**   Varicose veins are a recognised risk factor

☐   **D**   Oral combined contraceptive pill should be stopped before major surgery

☐   **E**   Calf vein thrombosis should be treated with heparin

SINGLE BEST ANSWER QUESTIONS

1   Select ONE of the following items about isolated systolic hypertension in the elderly

☐ **A**   Isolated systolic hypertension in the elderly effects between 15 and 20% of people over 60

☐ **B**   Isolated systolic hypertension confers no significant cardiovascular risk

☐ **C**   It is important to treat isolated systolic hypertension

☐ **D**   Diastolic blood pressure is a better predictor of risk than pulse pressure

2   The British Hypertension Society Guidelines recommend which ONE of the following?

☐ **A**   Adults should have their blood pressure checked every year

☐ **B**   Drug treatment is of proven value only until the age of 65 years

☐ **C**   Non-pharmacological advice is of borderline value

☐ **D**   Drug treatment should be tailored to the patient

☐ **E**   Few patients will need treatment from GPs

3   Select ONE of the following items about atrial fibrillation

☐ **A**   Atrial fibrillation is associated with a slight increase in the risk of stroke

☐ **B**   The risk associated with AF decreases with age

☐ **C**   Rate control is as important as rhythm control

☐ **D**   Patients have few concerns about taking warfarin

4   A high mortality following myocardial infarction is NOT associated with which ONE of the following?

☐ **A**   Increasing age

☐ **B**   High blood pressure

☐ **C**   High heart rate on admission to hospital

☐ **D**   Anterior infarction pattern on ECG

☐ **E**   Previous infarction

5   Select ONE of the following statements about angioplasty

☐ **A**   It is ideal for treatment of discrete stenosis of the main stem of the left coronary artery

☐ **B**   It is dangerous for patients with multiple vessel disease

☐ **C**   It is contraindicated in patients who have undergone bypass surgery

☐ **D**   It is contraindicated in patients with unstable angina

☐ **E**   It may involve complications if there is acute occlusion of the lesion

PHOTO QUESTION

THEME: CARDIOLOGY

For each ECG below, select the case history which is most likely to be seen in that patient.

1

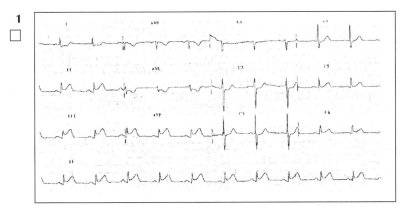

2

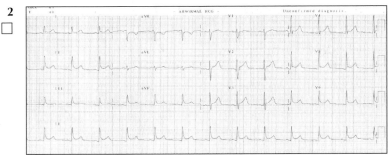

3

4

5

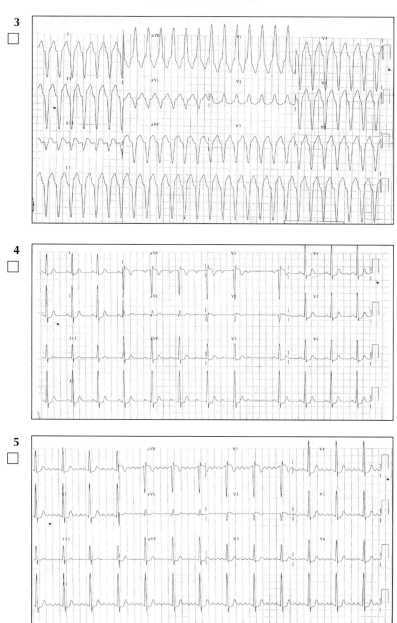

A   A 47-year-old man with 2-day history of retrosternal chest pain associated with a viral illness, relieved by leaning forward and aggravated by coughing.

B   A 55-year-old hypertensive company director who smokes 30 cigarettes a day who developed retrosternal chest pain during a board meeting.

C   A 72-year-old woman on the waiting list for mitral valve replacement complaining of palpitations.

D   A 76-year-old man six weeks post MI complains of shortness of breath; on examination he is hypotensive.

E   A 42-year-old man complaining of missed beats and a 2-week history of chest pain.

DERMATOLOGY/ENT/ OPHTHALMOLOGY

DERMATOLOGY

EXTENDED MATCHING QUESTIONS

THEME: RASHES

A Dermatitis artefacta

B Dermatitis herpetiformis

C Lichen simplex

D Nodular prurigo

For each of the descriptions, select the most likely rash. Each option may be used once, more than once, or not at all.

1 This rash characteristically has straight edges. ☐

2 If the itch/scratch cycle is interrupted then this lichenified rash disappears. ☐

3 This rash affects young adults. It is an itchy, vesicular rash with psoriatic distribution. ☐

4 This rash on the hands heals to leave white scars with follicular openings in them. ☐

THEME: CAUSES OF NAIL DISCOLORATION

A Chloroquine

B Leuconychia

C Penicillamine

D Tinea infection

E Trauma

F Yellow nail syndrome

For each description below, select the single most likely option. Each option may be used once, more than once, or not at all.

5 The nail is curved longitudinally and transversely and is associated with lymphoedema. ☐

6 The nails are stained yellow after taking certain medications. ☐

7 The nails are stained blue-grey. ☐

8 This is inherited as an autosomal dominant gene. ☐

9 The nails often have white streaks. ☐

10 There are yellow thickened areas with slow growth of the nail. ☐

11 The whole nail is white. ☐

THEME: RASHES

A Erythema multiforme

B Ichthyosis

C Infected eczema

D Pustular psoriasis

E Scabies

For each description below, select the single most likely diagnosis. Each option may be used once, more than once, or not at all.

12 This rash has secondary staphylococcal infection. ☐

13 There is scaly dry skin on the fingers. ☐

14 A large vesicle with a surrounding red halo is characteristic. ☐

15 Lesions are often seen on the soles of the feet and palms of the hand. ☐

16 Burrows occur on the sides of the fingers. ☐

THEME: LEG ULCERS

A Ischaemic ulcers

B Venous ulcers

For each description, select the most likely type of leg ulcer. Each option may be used once, more than once, or not at all.

17 Usually have marked induration and oedema. ☐

18 Usually painless and pigmented. ☐

19 Tend to be punched out and necrotic. ☐

20 Are painful and most frequently seen in elderly people. ☐

21 The surrounding skin may be eczematous. ☐

THEME: SKIN CONDITIONS

A   Allergic contact dermatitis

B   Asteatotic eczema

C   Atopic dermatitis

D   Erythrodermic psoriasis

E   Guttate psoriasis

F   Irritant contact dermatitis

G   Plaque psoriasis

H   Pompholyx

I   Pustular psoriasis

J   Seborrhoeic dermatitis

For each of the descriptions below, select the most appropriate diagnosis from the list above. Each option may be used once, more than once, or not at all.

22 Most commonly seen in children and adolescents; there are numerous small scaly papules and plaques.

23 Follows repeated exposure to an irritant, eg mineral oils in motor mechanics.

24 An eruption of vesicles on the sides of fingers, the palms or soles of the feet, which may be extremely itchy.

25 Also known as 'red man syndrome', this skin disease may affect the whole body and lead to hypothermia, hypoproteinaemia and high-output heart failure.

26 An erythematous condition, often with scaling in a characteristic crazy-paving pattern, seen on the shins of the elderly.

MULTIPLE BEST ANSWER QUESTIONS

1 **Which THREE of the following nail signs are suggestive of the associated conditions?**

- ☐ **A** Transverse grooves and psoriasis
- ☐ **B** Opaque nails and diabetes mellitus
- ☐ **C** Splinter haemorrhages and bacterial endocarditis
- ☐ **D** Blue nails and *Pseudomonas* spp. infection
- ☐ **E** Green nails and lichen planus

2 **Which TWO of the following skin conditions generally deteriorate during pregnancy?**

- ☐ **A** Atopic eczema
- ☐ **B** Systemic lupus erythematosus
- ☐ **C** Hidradenitis suppurativa
- ☐ **D** Herpes simplex

3 **Which TWO of the following drugs are characteristically linked with the following type of reaction?**

- ☐ **A** Oral contraceptives and photosensitivity
- ☐ **B** Codeine and urticaria
- ☐ **C** Tetracycline and exfoliative dermatitis
- ☐ **D** Fucidin® and pigmentation
- ☐ **E** Beta-blockers and eczema

4   Select THREE items which are true of granuloma annulare

☐ **A**   It is more common on the trunk

☐ **B**   It is painful

☐ **C**   It is associated with diabetes

☐ **D**   It may persist for many years

☐ **E**   It lacks effective treatment

5   Which TWO of the following conditions are associated with erythema nodosum?

☐ **A**   Herpes simplex

☐ **B**   Tuberculosis

☐ **C**   Inflammatory bowel disease

☐ **D**   Hyperthyroidism

6   Which TWO of the following drugs may precipitate or exacerbate psoriasis?

☐ **A**   Lithium

☐ **B**   Hydralazine

☐ **C** H_2 antagonists

☐ **D**   Beta-blockers

☐ **E**   Anticonvulsants

7   Select THREE of the following items concerning alopecia areata

☐ **A**   It is a scarring process with permanent loss of follicles

☐ **B**   It is associated with autoimmune thyroid disease

☐ **C**   It is confined to scalp hairs

☐ **D**   It is a recognised association of Down's syndrome

☐ **E**   It may be associated with nail changes

8   Select THREE of the following statements about acne vulgaris

☐ **A**   Most teenagers with acne seek treatment for it

☐ **B**   The key pathological event in acne is obstruction of the pilo-sebaceous duct

☐ **C**   The severity of acne is directly related to the degree of secretion of sebum

☐ **D**   Circulating levels of androgen are usually high in patients with acne

☐ **E**   An open comedo (blackhead) results from the rupture of the wall of the pilosebaceous duct and release of the contents in the dermis

SINGLE BEST ANSWER QUESTIONS

1   Select ONE of the following regarding basal cell carcinoma

☐   **A**   The most common skin malignancy in Caucasians

☐   **B**   Almost never occurs on covered skin sites

☐   **C**   Should no longer be treated by curettage and cautery since results are inferior to those of other treatment methods

2   Select ONE of the following regarding multiple seborrhoeic warts

☐   **A**   Most commonly found on the face and trunk

☐   **B**   Usually infective

☐   **C**   Best removed by excision

3   The ONE most recognised cause of erythema nodosum from the list below is

☐   **A**   Sarcoidosis

☐   **B**   Oral contraceptives

☐   **C**   Preceding *Mycoplasma* infection

4   You see a 6-year-old child in surgery with his mother. He has been diagnosed with molluscum contagiosum and she is keen to have him treated. Which ONE of the following is true?

☐   **A**   The condition resolves spontaneously

☐   **B**   The condition is not infectious

☐   **C**   Patients may treat themselves by squeezing the spots with no adverse effects

☐   **D**   It is only seen in children

☐   **E**   Piercing the lesions with an orange stick dipped in phenol is the treatment of choice

5   **You are setting up a leg ulcer clinic to be run by your practice nurse. Which ONE of the following is the single best treatment for venous leg ulcers?**

☐ **A**   Aspirin

☐ **B**   Compression bandaging

☐ **C**   Zinc paste

☐ **D**   Intermittent pneumatic calf compression

☐ **E**   Hyperbaric oxygen

PHOTO QUESTION

THEME: DERMATOLOGY

For each of the images below, select the most appropriate description from the selection.

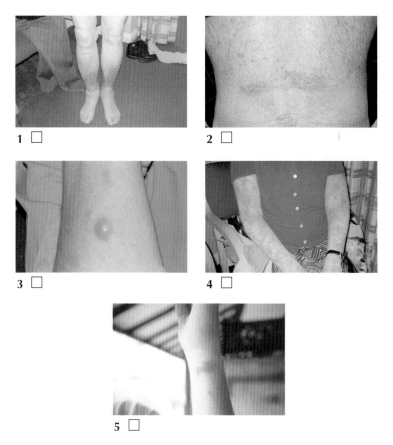

1 ☐

2 ☐

3 ☐

4 ☐

5 ☐

A Best treated with emollients, vitamin D analogues or ultraviolet light.

B Associated with characteristic macular skin lesions.

C A reaction to haemosiderin deposition.

D Irritation by plant sting.

E A phototoxic reaction seen after contact with plants.

ENT

EXTENDED MATCHING QUESTIONS

THEME: LESIONS ON THE EAR

A   Chilblains

B   Kerato-acanthoma

C   Psoriatic

D   Rodent ulcer

E   Squamous cell cancer

F   Tophi

For each of the descriptions, select the single most likely lesion. Each option may be used once, more than once, or not at all.

1 These lesions are common, painful and itchy.   □

2 This is a slow-growing lesion found on the helix.   □

3 These lesions are usually found on the antihelix.   □

4 These lesions are rapidly growing and usually found on the helix.   □

5 These lesions are usually found behind and below the ear.   □

6 These lesions are found in the external auditory meatus and on the skin behind and below the ear.   □

THEME: HOARSENESS

A   Diabetes mellitus

B   Gastro-oesophageal reflux

C   Myxoedema

D   Pharyngeal neoplasia

E   Smoking

F   Thyrotoxicosis

For each patient with hoarseness, select the single most likely diagnosis. Each option can be used once, more than once, or not at all.

7   Hoarseness with weight loss. ☐

8   Hoarseness in an otherwise healthy adult. ☐

9   Hoarseness with weight gain. ☐

10 Hoarseness with associated dysphagia. ☐

11 Hoarseness with dyspepsia. ☐

THEME: EARACHE

A   Otitis media

B   Otitis externa

C   Tonsillitis

D   Glue ear

E   Ménière's disease

F   Tonsillar carcinoma

G   Furuncle

H   Bullous haemorrhagic myringitis

I   Ramsay Hunt syndrome

J   Cerebellopontine angle tumours

For each of the descriptions below, select the most appropriate diagnosis from the list above. Each option may be used once, more than once, or not at all.

12 Earache associated with imbalance, deafness and vesicles in the ear canal. ☐

13 Peak incidence is around 6 years of age, this condition is the commonest cause of conductive hearing loss. ☐

14 Should be considered in patients with unilateral tinnitus, unsteadiness and deafness. ☐

15 May present with diarrhoea and vomiting in young children. ☐

16 May be caused by hearing aids. ☐

MULTIPLE BEST ANSWER QUESTIONS

1   Glue ear is commonly associated with which TWO of the following?

- ☐ **A** Atopy
- ☐ **B** Neomycin treatment
- ☐ **C** Breast-fed babies compared with bottle-fed
- ☐ **D** Meningitis
- ☐ **E** Down's syndrome

2   Which THREE of the following predispose to oral cancer?

- ☐ **A** High alcohol consumption
- ☐ **B** Smoking cigarettes
- ☐ **C** Folate deficiency
- ☐ **D** Tea drinking
- ☐ **E** Cigar smoking

3   Which THREE of the following factors predispose to otitis externa?

- ☐ **A** Ear syringing
- ☐ **B** Age under 5 years
- ☐ **C** Diabetes mellitus
- ☐ **D** Psoriasis
- ☐ **E** Diving

4   Which THREE of the following drugs cause a dry mouth?

☐ **A**   Monoamine oxidase inhibitors

☐ **B**   Antihistamines

☐ **C**   Bronchoconstrictors

☐ **D**   Phenothiazines

☐ **E**   Amphetamines

SINGLE BEST ANSWER QUESTIONS

1   Which ONE of the following is a recognised cause of conductive deafness in children?

☐ **A**   Glue ear

☐ **B**   Post-meningitis

☐ **C**   Congenital rubella

☐ **D**   Mumps

☐ **E**   Kernicterus

2   You see a 29-year-old policeman in surgery who complains of mild allergic rhinitis. Which ONE of the following is the best initial treatment?

☐ **A**   Referral for RAST testing for common allergens

☐ **B**   Oral desloratadine

☐ **C**   Nasal fluticasone on a prn basis

☐ **D**   Reduction to house dust mite exposure

☐ **E**   Chlorphenamine (chlorpheniramine)

☐ **F**   Regular xylometazoline

3   A 72-year-old man is brought to see you by his wife who says she is sick of having to shout every time she wants to talk to him. An audiogram confirms sensorineural deafness. Which ONE of the following is the likeliest cause?

☐ **A**   Otosclerosis

☐ **B**   Multiple sclerosis

☐ **C**   Barotrauma

☐ **D**   Presbyacusis

☐ **E**   Ménière's disease

PHOTO QUESTION

THEME: AUDIOGRAMS

For each audiogram shown below, select the most appropriate phrase from the list below.

A   Noise-induced hearing loss.

B   Presbyacusis.

C   Normal.

D   Severe bilateral hearing loss.

E   Severe unilateral hearing loss.

1

☐

2

☐

3

☐

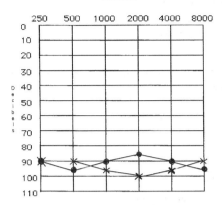

4

☐

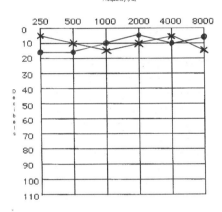

5

☐

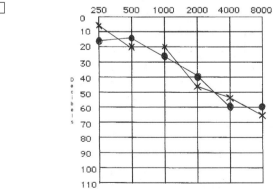

OPHTHALMOLOGY

EXTENDED MATCHING QUESTIONS

THEME: SUDDEN LOSS OF VISION

A Central retinal vein occlusion

B Migraine

C Optic neuritis

D Senile macular degeneration

E Toxic optic neuropathy

For each description, select the single most likely cause of sudden loss of vision. Each option may be used once, more than once, or not at all.

1 There is a gradual loss of vision in people between 20 and 45 years old. The peripheral vision is intact. ☐

2 There is a gradually progressive loss of vision in an older person. There is preservation of peripheral fields. ☐

3 This tends to occur in heavy cigarette smokers. Peripheral vision remains largely intact. ☐

4 There is complete recovery from this loss of vision which often, but not always, occurs with headache. ☐

5 There is extensive haemorrhage visible into the fundus. Visual loss develops over a few hours. ☐

THEME: RED EYE

A Acute glaucoma

B Episcleritis

C Iritis

D Keratitis

E Subconjunctival haemorrhage

For each description, select the single most likely cause of red eye. Each option may be used once, more than once, or not at all.

6 This is associated with impaired vision; an ulcer may be found near the visual axis. ☐

7 There is slight or no pain; vision tends to be normal and the red eye will settle without treatment. ☐

8 The pupil is small and often distorted. ☐

9 There is severe pain with severe visual impairment; vomiting commonly occurs. ☐

10 This red eye is painless and vision is normal. ☐

THEME: VISUAL FIELD DEFECTS

A Arcuate scotoma

B Central scotoma

C Centrocaecal scotoma

D Ring scotoma

For each description, select the single most likely visual field defect. Each option may be used once, more than once, or not at all.

11 This is characteristic of glaucoma. ☐

12 This field defect occurs in toxic neuropathy. ☐

13 This scotoma is typical of retinitis pigmentosa. ☐

14 This defect is characteristic of disease affecting the macula. ☐

THEME: EYE LESIONS

A   Corneal arcus

B   Kayser–Fleischer rings

C   Pinguecula

D   Pterygium

E   Subconjunctival haemorrhage

For each description, select the single most likely eye lesion. Each option may be used once, more than once, or not at all.

15 A triangular fold of conjunctiva found between the canthus and the corneal edge. ☐

16 A white ring found near the outer margin of the cornea. ☐

17 A bright red mark seen on the conjunctiva. ☐

18 A yellowish-brown deposit seen at the periphery of the cornea. ☐

19 A yellow deposit noted between the canthus and the edge of the cornea. ☐

20 Due to a deposit of copper. ☐

21 May occur as a result of whooping cough or labour. ☐

MULTIPLE BEST ANSWER QUESTIONS

1   Select TWO from the following list as features of acute iritis

☐   **A**   Dilated pupil

☐   **B**   Circumcorneal redness

☐   **C**   Blurred vision

☐   **D**   Purulent discharge

☐   **E**   Hard and tender eye

2   Select TWO findings in myopia

☐   **A**   Minus (concave) lenses are required in the ophthalmoscope to view the fundus

☐   **B**   The optic disc may look small

☐   **C**   The optic disc may look particularly bright

☐   **D**   There may be surrounding chorioretinal atrophy

3   Select FOUR of the following statements about ocular fundus findings

☐   **A**   Hard exudates are caused by sugars leaking out of blood vessels

☐   **B**   Hard exudates are seen in diabetes and hypertension

☐   **C**   Hard exudates look like deposits of cotton wool

☐   **D**   Soft exudates are due to swelling of the axons in the nerve fibre layer

☐   **E**   Soft exudates are well-defined yellow-white deposits, often in rings

☐   **F**   Soft exudates occur around an area of infarcted retina

☐   **G**   Soft exudates are often associated with features of retinal ischaemia, such as new blood vessel formation

SINGLE BEST ANSWER QUESTIONS

1 What is the commonest cause of blindness over the age of 65 years?

- ☐ **A** Glaucoma
- ☐ **B** Cataract
- ☐ **C** Diabetic retinopathy
- ☐ **D** Macular degeneration

2 What is the commonest cause of blindness in people aged 45–64?

- ☐ **A** Diabetic retinopathy
- ☐ **B** Macular degeneration
- ☐ **C** Glaucoma
- ☐ **D** Optic atrophy

3 Cataracts are NOT usually associated with

- ☐ **A** myotonic dystrophy
- ☐ **B** thyrotoxicosis
- ☐ **C** diabetes mellitus
- ☐ **D** rubella
- ☐ **E** hyperparathyroidism

4 Select ONE statement. Diabetic maculopathy

- ☐ **A** is more common in NIDDM than in IDDM
- ☐ **B** impairs peripheral vision
- ☐ **C** is treated by panretinal photocoagulation
- ☐ **D** is characterised by drusen at the macula
- ☐ **E** causes painful visual loss

5   A patient presents with a painful red eye. Which ONE of the
    following findings is more suggestive of acute conjunctivitis than
    anterior uveitis?

☐   **A**   Blurring of vision

☐   **B**   Profuse discharge

☐   **C**   Small pupil

☐   **D**   Photophobia

PHOTO QUESTION

THEME: OPHTHALMOLOGY

For each retinal photo below, select the description of symptoms most likely to be associated with this photo.

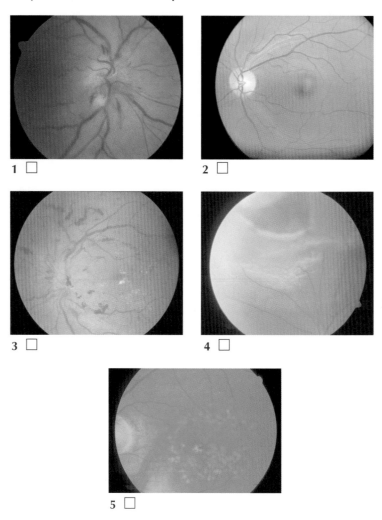

1 ☐

2 ☐

3 ☐

4 ☐

5 ☐

A   A 54-year-old type 1 diabetic with neuropathy and nephropathy.

B   A 60-year-old myope who complains of an episode of flashing lights in his right eye followed by a reduction in his peripheral vision when he closes his left eye.

C   A 72-year-old with general malaise over several months with a 12-hour history of severe temporal headache and tenderness; the other retina is normal.

D   An 84-year-old complaining of increasing difficulty reading and distortion of straight lines.

E   A 64-year-old with severe osteoarthritis in both knees.

ENDOCRINOLOGY/METABOLIC

EXTENDED MATCHING QUESTIONS

THEME: OSTEOPOROSIS

A   Bisphosphonates

B   Calcitonin

C   Calcium and vitamin D

D   Corticosteroids

E   Family history

F   Hip protectors

G   Hormone replacement therapy (HRT)

H   Obesity

I   Parathyroid hormone

J   Smoking, drinking and exercise

Choose one of the above options for each of the following statements.

1   Effective in reducing the impact of falls. ☐

2   Can cause a fall in bone mass and bone density. ☐

3   Recommended by NICE to treat post-menopausal women with severe osteoporosis. ☐

4   The treatment of choice for preventing osteoporosis in women under 50 who have had a premature menopause. ☐

5   Once this treatment has been stopped for 10 years, bone density and fracture risk are similar with or without this treatment. ☐

6   The Committee for the Safety of Medicines advise this is no longer the treatment of choice for preventing osteoporosis in women over the age of 50. ☐

7   Is an irreversible risk factor for osteoporosis. ☐

THEME: ENDOCRINE DISEASES

A Acromegaly

B Conn's syndrome

C Cushing's syndrome

D Diabetes insipidus

E Simmond's disease

For each of the descriptions, select the most likely endocrine disease. Each option may be used once, more than once, or not at all.

8 Caused by excess growth hormone. ☐

9 Caused by a deficiency of antidiuretic hormone (ADH). ☐

10 Associated with excess corticosteroid. ☐

11 Associated with excess aldosterone. ☐

12 Associated with deficiencies of growth hormone (GH), follicle-stimulating hormone (FSH) and luteinising hormone (LH). ☐

THEME: METABOLIC BONE DISEASE

A   Hyperparathyroidism

B   Hypoparathyroidism

C   Osteomalacia

D   Osteoporosis

E   Paget's disease

F   Renal osteodystrophy

G   Rickets

For each of the descriptions, select the most likely metabolic bone disease. Each option may be used once, more than once, or not at all.

13 Associated with a greatly increased alkaline phosphatase level, bone pain and tenderness; the sacrum and lumbar spine are the bones most commonly affected.

14 Children present with leg and chest deformities; it is associated with increased alkaline phosphatase and decreased phosphate levels.

15 Presents with bone pain and tenderness and is associated with a moderate increase in alkaline phosphatase levels, and decreased phosphate and calcium levels.

16 Associated with decreased calcium levels but increased phosphate levels.

17 This disease can be complicated by progressive occlusion of skull foramina, causing deafness, and also by high-output cardiac failure.

18 Associated with increased calcium levels, bone cysts and subperiosteal erosions in the phalanges.

19 This causes cupping, splaying and fraying of the epiphyses.

20 Hormone replacement therapy is given to try to avoid this disease.

THEME: ARTHRITIS

A Ankylosing spondylitis

B Dysbaric osteonecrosis

C Gout

D Primary nodal osteoarthritis

E Pseudogout

F Psoriatic arthritis

G Reiter's syndrome

H Rheumatic fever

I Rheumatoid arthritis

J Rubella

K Septic arthritis

L Systemic lupus erythematosus

Read the case summaries below and select the most appropriate diagnosis from the list above. Each option may be used once, more than once, or not at all.

21 A 37-year-old man with history of backache over several years, which disturbs his sleep. He has early morning stiffness, which improves with exercise.

22 A 19-year-old sewage worker presents with bilateral knee pain and stiffness. He also mentions red spots on his feet that are turning into pustules. These symptoms started a few days after an episode of gastroenteritis.

23 A 45-year-old accountant complains of recurrent pain in the ends of his fingers and toes. He tells you that it seems to get worse when his skin is dry and he has thickened distorted nails on the affected fingers.

24 A 21-year-old woman presents with fever and rigors. She has also developed a swollen, red and painful knee.

25 A 44-year-old man with mild hypertension, recently started on diuretics, wakes up in the middle of the night with severe pain in his big toe. On examination the skin overlying the joint is red, swollen and warm.

26 A 4-year-old child who has been unwell for several days with coryzal symptoms and conjunctivitis develops a rash, initially on his face but spreading to his trunk. He subsequently complains of pain and stiffness in his metacarpophalangeal and proximal interphalangeal joints.

MULTIPLE BEST ANSWER QUESTIONS

1   Choose THREE statements about gout

☐   **A**   Predominantly affects males

☐   **B**   Is usually, but not always, accompanied by elevated serum uric acid levels

☐   **C**   Is associated with high alcohol intake, due to the high purine content of alcoholic drinks

☐   **D**   Is closely associated with potassium-sparing diuretics

☐   **E**   Can cause renal impairment

2   Hyperuricaemia may be induced by which THREE of the following?

☐   **A**   Furosemide (frusemide)

☐   **B**   Polycythaemia rubra vera

☐   **C**   Myxoedema

☐   **D**   Multiple myeloma

☐   **E**   Diabetes mellitus

3   Which of the following THREE conditions are recognised causes of fasting hypoglycaemia?

☐   **A**   Lung cancer

☐   **B**   Alcoholism

☐   **C**   Addison's disease

☐   **D**   Hepatic carcinoma

☐   **E**   Chronic gout

☐   **F**   Myxoedema

4   THREE recognised complications in pregnancies of diabetic women are

☐ **A**   Oligohydramnios

☐ **B**   Pre-eclampsia

☐ **C**   Congenital abnormalities

☐ **D**   Intra-uterine growth retardation

☐ **E**   Intra-uterine death

SINGLE BEST ANSWER QUESTIONS

1   Which ONE of the following confirms the diagnosis of diabetes mellitus, in a patient with polyuria, thirst and weight loss?

☐   **A**   Random glucose greater or equal to 11.1 mmol/l

☐   **B**   Fasting glucose greater or equal to 6.0 mmol/l

☐   **C**   Glucose greater or equal to 9.1 mmol/l two hours after 75 g of glucose in an oral glucose tolerance test

2   Which ONE of the following is not a standard of the NSF for diabetes mellitus?

☐   **A**   Identification of people with diabetes mellitus

☐   **B**   Empowering people with diabetes mellitus

☐   **C**   Clinical care of children with diabetes mellitus

☐   **D**   Clinical care of adults with diabetes mellitus

☐   **E**   Management of diabetic emergencies

☐   **F**   Prevention of type 1 diabetes mellitus

3   Which ONE of the following does NOT occur in hypothyroidism?

☐   **A**   Carpal tunnel syndrome

☐   **B**   Pretibial myxoedema

☐   **C**   Macrocytosis

☐   **D**   A normal serum triiodothyronine (T_3) concentration

4 Carpal tunnel syndrome is NOT usually associated with which ONE of the following?

☐ **A** Pregnancy

☐ **B** Rheumatoid arthritis

☐ **C** Thyrotoxicosis

☐ **D** Previous scaphoid fracture

☐ **E** Acromegaly

SUMMARY COMPLETION QUESTION

THEME: TYPE 2 DIABETES MANAGEMENT

As a result of the new GMS contract you are reviewing the management of type 2 diabetes mellitus. It has been suggested that you refer all patients at diagnosis to a dietician for advice on diet and lipids. Consider the following extract from a trial of this approach and the summary below, choosing appropriate options from the list for each gap in the summary.

Fat intake in patients newly diagnosed with type 2 diabetes: a 4-year follow-up study in general practice. Van de Laar *et al* British Journal of General Practitioners 2004;54:177–82.

Abstract

Background Although treatment targets for the consumption of dietary fat in patients with type 2 diabetes mellitus are well accepted, little is known about the actual fat consumption by newly diagnosed patients or the dietary adjustments that they make in the following years.

Aims To measure fat intake in patients with type 2 diabetes mellitus in general practice at diagnosis, shortly after dietary consultation, and after 4 years.

Design of study A prospective cohort study.

Setting Thirty-three general practices in the Netherlands.

Method One hundred and forty-four patients with newly diagnosed type 2 diabetes mellitus were referred to a dietician, and fat consumption (the main outcome measure) was assessed with a 104-item food frequency questionnaire at diagnosis, 8 weeks following diagnosis and after 4 years. Reference values for fat consumption were obtained from an age-matched sample of a population-based survey.

Results At diagnosis, total energy intake was 10.6 MJ/day and cholesterol intake was 300 mg/day. Total fat consumption was 40.9% of energy intake, with saturated fatty acids 15.0%, monounsaturated fatty acids 14.3%, and polyunsaturated fatty acids 9.2% of energy intake. All levels, except for polyunsaturated fatty acids, were significantly unfavourable compared with those for the general population. After 8 weeks, consumption of saturated fatty acids had decreased to a lower level than in the general population and all other levels measured were similar to those for the general population. After 4 years there was a slight increase in the consumption of total fat and monounsaturated fatty acids, but cholesterol and saturated fatty acid consumption had decreased further.

Conclusions Patients with newly diagnosed type 2 diabetes mellitus have an unfavourable fat consumption at diagnosis. They adapt to a more desirable consumption shortly after diagnosis, and this improved dietary behaviour is sustained for 4 years. Recommendations regarding consumption of total and saturated fat are, in contrast to those for cholesterol, not met by patients in general practice.

Table 2 Changes in consumption of total energy and fat by patients newly diagnosed with type 2 diabetes mellitus: mean changes from diagnosis to 8 weeks, from diagnosis to 4 years, and from 8 weeks to 4 years. A negative value indicates a decrease in time.

	Change in mean difference (95% CI)		
	From diagnosis to 8 weeks[a]	From diagnosis to 4 years[b]	From 8 weeks to 4 years[c]
Energy intake (MJ/day)	−2.2 (−2.6 to −1.7)	−1.8 (−2.3 to −1.2)	0.5[d] (0.09 to 0.9)
Total fat (En%)	−5.1 (−6.6 to −3.5)	−3.0 (−4.8 to −1.2)	2.5 (1.1 to 3.9)
Saturated fatty acids (En%)	−2.4 (−3.0 to −1.8)	−3.1 (−3.8 to −2.3)	−0.5[d] (−1.1 to 0.1)
Monounsaturated fatty acids (En%)	−2.5 (−3.1 to −1.8)	−1.5 (−2.3 to −0.6)	1.0 (0.4 to 1.6)
Polyunsaturated fatty acids (En%)	0.3[d] (−0.4 to 0.9)	0.9[d] (0.0 to 1.7)	0.9[d] (0.0 to 1.8)
Cholesterol intake (mg/day)	−63.1 (−77.8 to −48.3)	−99.7 (−120.0 to −79.4)	−33.6 (−48.3 to −18.8)
Cholesterol intake (mg/MJ)	−0.3[d] (−1.5 to 1.0)	−6.2 (−7.8 to −4.6)	−5.6 (−7.2 to −4.0)

[a]($n = 110$), [b]($n = 106$), [c]($n = 86$), [d]All values except these are significant ($P<0.0024$). Significance tests are done with an α of 0.0024 (0.05:21) in order to account for multiple testing. En% = % of energy intake.

Summary

This study is a____**(1)**____cohort study which assigned all newly diagnosed diabetics to the intervention of referral to a dietician. The dietician followed a standardised programme of two consultation sessions offering advice tailored to the patients' individual needs. All dieticians were registered, but there is no information given to confirm that they were all following standard advice, nor whether any of them had a special interest in diabetes. The prospective cohort design of the study does not allow comparison with____**(2)**____.

The study did not look at clinical outcomes such as morbidity, but used ____**(3)**____ outcomes to obtain meaningful data within the timescale of the study. The results in Table 2 show that the intervention resulted in a significant ____**(4)**____ in total energy intake, total fat, and cholesterol at 8 weeks, maintained at 4 years. For each of these the reductions were statistically significant, with the 95% confidence intervals confirming this. *P* values were ____**(5)**____0.05, confirming statistical significance. There was also a significant decrease in ____**(6)**____ confirming improved control.

Overall these results are encouraging. Several questions are however raised which must be considered before adopting the policy. Firstly, in the absence of a control group receiving normal care, is there any evidence that the outcomes are any better than would otherwise be expected? A diagnosis of diabetes is a ____**(7)**____ motivator for change and may in itself result in significant lifestyle change. Other potential ____**(8)**____ influences include potential variability in the intervention: no standardised protocols were used and there may be differences in the experience and approach of the dieticians.

Options

A   Reduction

B   Confounding

C   >

D   Surrogate

E   Powerful

F   Increase

G   Controls

H   Prospective

I   Polyunsaturated fatty acids

J   <

K   Decrease

L   Distracting

M   Weak

N   HbA1c

O   Retrospective

SUMMARY COMPLETION QUESTION

THEME: DIABETES AND COGNITIVE DECLINE

One of your diabetic patients tells you that she has heard that diabetes causes dementia. You agree to look into this and come across the following paper. Read the extract and then the summary below, selecting the appropriate response for each gap.

Prospective study of type 2 diabetes and cognitive decline in women aged 70–81 years. Logroscino *et al* British Medical Journal 2004;328:548–51.

Methods

The Nurses' Health Study is a prospective cohort of 121, 700 US female registered nurses, who were aged 30–55 years in 1976, when the study began. Participants' health information has been updated with biennial mailed questionnaires. Over 90% of the original cohort have been followed up to date.

From 1995 to 2001, participants aged 70 years and older who had not had a stroke were given baseline cognitive assessments by telephone. Overall, 93% completed the interview. Interviewers were blinded to participants' health status (including diabetes). For the baseline analyses of cognitive function, we included 18, 999 women with complete information on education and without type 1 diabetes, gestational diabetes, or unconfirmed diabetes (see below).

The follow-up cognitive assessment began about two years after the baseline interview. After the exclusion of the 3% who died, calls have been attempted for 98% to date. Of these, 92% (*n* = 16, 596) completed the interview, 5% (*n* = 967) refused, 3% (*n* = 526) were unreachable. For analyses of cognitive decline, we included 16, 596 participants who completed both assessments and excluded women in whom diabetes had been newly diagnosed between the baseline and second interviews.

Assessment of cognitive function

Our cognitive assessment has been previously described. Briefly, we initially administered only the telephone interview for cognitive status (TICS) (n = 18, 999) but gradually added more tests: immediate (n = 18, 295) and delayed recalls of the East Boston memory test (n = 18, 268), test of verbal fluency (naming animals, n = 18, 285), digit span backwards (n = 16, 591), and delayed recall of a 10-word list (n = 16, 582). To summarise performance, we calculated a global score averaging results of the six tests using z scores (16, 563 women completed all six tests).

Ascertainment of type 2 diabetes

We identified women who reported that diabetes had been diagnosed by a physician before the baseline cognitive interview. We then confirmed reports based on responses to a supplementary questionnaire including complications, diagnostic tests and treatment; confirmations conformed to guidelines of the National Diabetes Data Group until 1997, and revised criteria of the American Diabetes Association from 1998. Validation studies found 98% concordance of our nurse participants' reports of type 2 diabetes with medical records. We estimated duration of diabetes by subtracting date of diagnosis from date of baseline cognitive interview. We obtained information on recent drug treatment for diabetes from the biennial questionnaire before the baseline interview.

Statistical analyses

Potential confounding factors – data on potential confounders were identified from information provided as of the questionnaire immediately before the baseline cognitive assessment. All potential confounding variables were selected a priori based on risk factors for cognitive function in the existing literature (see Tables 3 and 4). In analyses of cognitive decline, we adjusted for baseline performance.

Summary

Diabetes and its complications represent one of the greatest public health challenges of the 21st century. As the true scale of the epidemic becomes apparent, the importance of good control to prevent complications has become one of our top priorities. This paper looks at both the____(1)____of diabetes and cognitive decline and the impact of diabetic control on____(2)____.

The subjects are drawn from the Nurses' Health Study, a prospective cohort study of 18, 999 women. This large pool of subjects lends the study significant____**(3)**____which should facilitate demonstration of small effects. The subjects represent a____**(4)**____socioeconomic spectrum, and are all presumably educated to college level. This will tend to____**(5)**____confounding influences such as baseline IQ which may effect functioning in the cognitive assessment. No apparent attempts have been made to control other potential contributors such as smoking, Alzheimer's or uncontrolled hypertension. The assessments were based on a standardised, validated tool, minimising observer bias.

The authors have attempted to ensure that there is____**(6)**____in the diagnosis of diabetes, and followed up volunteered information of a diagnosis with examination of their medical record to confirm the diagnosis. This should ensure that the patients in the diabetic group do indeed have diabetes. Unfortunately the authors have not made any such effort to screen the control group for____**(7)**____diabetes. Diabetes is often undiagnosed and patients may present with complications of diabetes. Thus failure to control for this factor____**(8)**____differences between the groups and thus the association between diabetes and cognitive decline.

Options

A	Reduce	**N**	Consistency
B	Narrow	**O**	Concordance
C	Reduces	**P**	Uniformity
D	Outcomes		
E	Wide		
F	Increases		
G	Association		
H	Latent		
I	Power		
J	Pathology		
K	Undiagnosed		
L	Increase		
M	Strengthens		

PHOTO QUESTION

THEME: HANDS

For each image, select the case description which is most likely to correspond to the history.

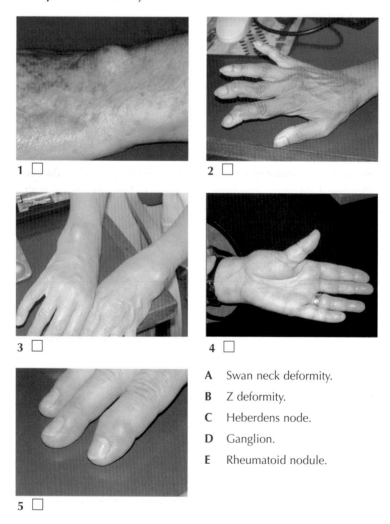

1 ☐

2 ☐

3 ☐

4 ☐

A   Swan neck deformity.

B   Z deformity.

C   Heberdens node.

D   Ganglion.

E   Rheumatoid nodule.

5 ☐

GASTROENTEROLOGY/NUTRITION

EXTENDED MATCHING QUESTIONS

THEME: CAUSES OF ABDOMINAL PAIN

A   Appendicitis

B   Cholecystitis

C   Crohn's disease

D   Diverticular disease

E   Irritable bowel syndrome

F   Ischaemic colitis

G   Pancreatitis

For each of the following scenarios, select the most appropriate diagnostic option. Each option may be used once, more than once, or not at all.

1   A 41-year-old restaurant manager who has severe abdominal pain radiating to his back. ☐

2   A 72-year-old lady who has 'life-long' constipation and has had vague abdominal pain for months or even years; she is tender in her left lower abdomen. ☐

3   A 31-year-old doctor who has abdominal pain relieved by defaecation, she has frequent loose motions, often after meals; she is tender over her sigmoid colon. ☐

4   A 69-year-old lady with abdominal pain and bloody diarrhoea; she has frequent angina; her abdomen is generally tender. ☐

5   A 58-year-old female teacher with feelings of 'fullness' and alternating diarrhoea and constipation; the pain is often relieved by passing flatus; she is tender in the left iliac fossa. ☐

6   A 49-year-old architect who has abdominal pain that he finds difficult to place, but says it is severe at times; his abdomen is generally tender, especially over the upper quadrants. ☐

7   A 41-year-old librarian with abdominal pain and diarrhoea; his abdomen is generally tender and he is noted to have anal tags. ☐

THEME: CHANGE IN BOWEL HABIT

A   Carcinoid syndrome

B   Coeliac disease

C   Colon cancer

D   Crohn's disease

E   Giardiasis

F   Hyperthyroidism

G   Irritable bowel syndrome

H   Laxative abuse

I   Toddler diarrhoea

J   Ulcerative colitis

K   Viral gastroenteritis

For each of the scenarios described below, pick the single most likely diagnosis. Each answer may be used once, more than once, or not at all.

8 The patient is systemically well; stools often contain undigested food, such as peas or carrots. ☐

9 Typically presents in the third to fourth decade with altered bowel habit, pain and bloating; commoner in women than men and symptoms do not usually disturb sleep. ☐

10 Causes bloody diarrhoea, up to ten times a day; relapses may be associated with stopping smoking. ☐

11 Characteristically causes flushing provoked by stress or alcohol; the diarrhoea is associated with weight loss, dyspnoea and wheezing. ☐

12 May be associated with increased appetite, palpitations, weight loss, anxiety and sweating. ☐

13 May present in childhood as failure to thrive, or in adults with diarrhoea, lethargy and malaise; may have an associated itchy vesicular rash. ☐

14 Characterised by an acute onset of anorexia, nausea, abdominal distension and frequent frothy yellow offensive stools. ☐

THEME: INDIGESTION

A Alginates

B Calcium carbonate

C Cisapride

D Domperidone

E H_2-receptor antagonist

F Misoprostol

G Nissen's fundoplication

H Proton pump inhibitor

I Triple therapy

For each of the clinical situations described below, select the most appropriate treatment from the list above. Each option may be used once, more than once, or not at all.

15 The first-line treatment for reflux in pregnancy. ☐

16 Should be considered in patients shown to have erosive oesophagitis on endoscopy. ☐

17 May be used in combination with NSAIDs to prevent ulcer formation. ☐

18 Should be considered for refractory reflux disease. ☐

19 The first-line treatment for *Helicobacter pylori*-positive patients with reflux symptoms whose symptoms are not helped by alginates. ☐

MULTIPLE BEST ANSWER QUESTIONS

1   Select TWO of the following statements about gallstones

☐ **A**   Cholesterol stones are strongly associated with bacteria in the bile

☐ **B**   The incidence of stones in the gall bladder rises with age

☐ **C**   Few stones remain symptomless

☐ **D**   Treatment with chenodeoxycholic acid may be effective for pigment stones

☐ **E**   Cholecystectomy is the standard treatment for symptomatic gallstones

2   Select TWO of the following items concerning *Helicobacter pylori*

☐ **A**   Infection is usually acquired in the first five years of life

☐ **B**   Is found in 50% of those over 50 years in developed countries

☐ **C**   Is strongly associated with gastro-oesophageal reflux

☐ **D**   Infection rate is increasing with improved socioeconomic conditions

☐ **E**   Breath test remains positive for about six months after eradication treatment

3   Select TWO of the following items about acute gastroenteritis

☐ **A**   Patients with an ileostomy are at increased risk of dehydration

☐ **B**   Refeeding should commence as soon as the appetite returns

☐ **C**   Oral rehydration therapy (ORT) improves the diarrhoea

☐ **D**   Antibiotics are contraindicated with *Campylobacter* infection

☐ **E**   Commercial ORT is inadequate for children under 2 years of age

4   Which TWO of the following are recognised complications of Crohn's disease?

☐ **A**   Small bowel obstruction

☐ **B**   Clubbing

☐ **C**   Polycythaemia

☐ **D**   Thrombophlebitis

☐ **E**   Amyloidosis

5   Select TWO of these statements about peptic ulceration

☐ **A**   Is associated with *H. pylori* infection in more than 90% of the cases

☐ **B**   Endoscopy is an essential diagnostic test

☐ **C**   In case of duodenal ulceration, pain is related to hunger

☐ **D**   Vomiting associated with pain is a diagnostic feature

☐ **E** H_2 antagonists have a place in the treatment

6   Select TWO of the following statements about duodenal ulceration

☐ **A**   Usually occurs in the duodenal bulb

☐ **B**   Affects approximately 10% of the population

☐ **C**   Has been proved to be caused by non-steroidal anti-inflammatory drugs

☐ **D**   Has a natural history of settling spontaneously within 5–10 years of onset

☐ **E**   Causes pain with a characteristic history of occurring immediately after food

7   In cancer of the colon, which THREE statements apply?

☐ **A** The overall 5-year survival rate is now about 50%

☐ **B** There is an increased risk in patients with inflammatory bowel disease

☐ **C** There is greater risk in patients with a family history of non-polyposis coli colonic cancer

☐ **D** There is an increased risk in patients who have two first-degree relatives with colonic cancer

☐ **E** Screening for faecal occult blood has a high sensitivity but a low specificity

8   Select THREE statements concerning diverticular disease of the colon

☐ **A** Is less common in vegetarians

☐ **B** Is commonly limited to the sigmoid colon

☐ **C** In General Practice, change in bowel habit is the most common presentation

☐ **D** Symptomatic diverticulosis needs treatment with a high-fibre diet

☐ **E** Acute diverticulitis is a common complication

9   Regarding colorectal cancer, in a 60-year-old man which TWO of the following symptoms/signs require urgent referral?

☐ **A** Change in bowel habit, decreasing frequency of defaecation

☐ **B** Rectal bleeding with anal symptoms

☐ **C** Lower abdominal pain without evidence of intestinal obstruction

☐ **D** Hb < 11 g/dl

☐ **E** Abdominal mass in the right iliac fossa

SINGLE BEST ANSWER QUESTIONS

1   Which ONE of the following is least likely to be associated with jaundice?

☐   **A**   Arsenic

☐   **B**   Methyldopa

☐   **C**   Atenolol

☐   **D**   Chlorpromazine

☐   **E**   Oral contraceptive pill

2   Select ONE statement. Ultrasound examination of the biliary system

☐   **A**   is as accurate as oral cholecystography in demonstrating gall bladder calculi

☐   **B**   will demonstrate the cause of bile duct obstruction in only 25% of cases

☐   **C**   cannot diagnose biliary carcinoma

☐   **D**   yields approximately 50% false-negative results in differentiating bile duct obstruction from non-obstructive jaundice

☐   **E**   cannot be performed in the fasting patient

3   Select ONE statement. Irritable bowel syndrome

☐   **A**   may follow an episode of infective diarrhoea

☐   **B**   is a diagnosis which can only be safely made following a normal colonoscopy or barium enema

☐   **C**   is commonly found to have been present in early adult life in patients presenting with diverticular disease in middle age

☐   **D**   rarely presents over the age of 60

4 **Which ONE of the following drugs does not cause constipation?**

☐ **A** Aluminium trisilicate

☐ **B** Tricyclic antidepressants

☐ **C** Oral contraceptives

☐ **D** Cimetidine

☐ **E** Iron

5 **Select ONE of the following items concerning irritable bowel syndrome**

☐ **A** Is more common in women than in men

☐ **B** Often presents in middle to old age

☐ **C** Causes abdominal pain made worse by defaecation

☐ **D** Causes rectal bleeding

☐ **E** Seldom affects children

6 **Which ONE of the following statements concerning diverticular disease is correct?**

☐ **A** Often occurs without symptoms

☐ **B** Affects the transverse colon more commonly than the sigmoid colon

☐ **C** Commonly presents with rectal bleeding

☐ **D** Should not be treated with morphine as this increases muscle spasm

☐ **E** Usually requires immediate surgery

PHOTO QUESTION

THEME: MISCELLANEOUS

For each image select the most appropriate initial treatment from the list below. Use each option only once.

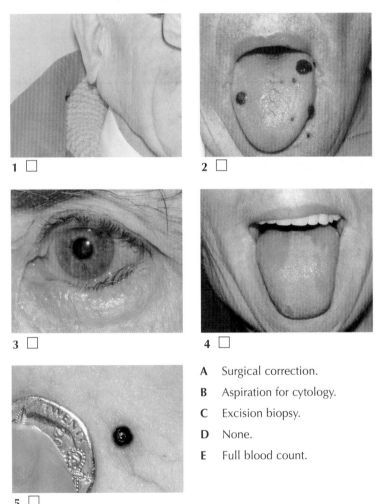

1 ☐

2 ☐

3 ☐

4 ☐

A Surgical correction.

B Aspiration for cytology.

C Excision biopsy.

D None.

E Full blood count.

5 ☐

INFECTIOUS DISEASES/ HAEMATOLOGY/IMMUNOLOGY/ ALLERGIES/GENETICS

EXTENDED MATCHING QUESTIONS

THEME: TREATMENT OF INFLUENZA

A   Broad spectrum antibiotics

B   Co-trimoxazole

C   Erythromycin

D   Neuraminidase inhibitors

E   Oseltamivir

F   Retroviral agents

G   Vaccination

H   Zanamivir

Choose one of the above options for each of the following statements. Each option may be used once, more than once or not at all.

1 Clinically effective for the treatment of influenza in otherwise healthy adults. ☐

2 When taken as prophylaxis decrease the likelihood of developing influenza by over 70%. ☐

3 The most important measure for reducing mortality in high-risk groups. ☐

4 The most important measure for reducing morbidity in high-risk groups. ☐

5 Recommended by NICE for the treatment of at-risk adults when influenza is in the community and the patient presents within 36 hours of developing symptoms. ☐

6 Has to be taken as an inhaler or nasal spray. ☐

THEME: CHROMOSOME DISORDERS

A Autosomal dominant

B Autosomal recessive

C X-linked

For each of the following conditions, select the type of chromosome disorder from the list above. Each option may be used once, more than once, or not at all.

  7 Haemophilia A. ☐

  8 Familial hypercholesterolaemia. ☐

  9 Cystic fibrosis. ☐

10 Red–green colour blindness. ☐

11 Familial polyposis coli. ☐

THEME: INFECTIVE AGENTS ASSOCIATED WITH TUMOURS

A   Epstein–Barr virus

B   *Helicobacter pylori*

C   Hepatitis B virus

D   Human herpesvirus type 8

E   Human papillomavirus

F   Measles virus

G   Parvovirus

For each of the following tumours, select the infective agent associated with the tumour from the list above. Each option may be used once, more than once, or not at all.

12 Gastric lymphoma. ☐

13 Hepatocellular carcinoma. ☐

14 Kaposi's sarcoma. ☐

15 Genital warts. ☐

16 Squamous cell carcinoma of cervix. ☐

MULTIPLE BEST ANSWER QUESTIONS

1 Which TWO of the following are NOT typical features of Turner's syndrome?

☐ **A** XY genotype

☐ **B** Tall stature

☐ **C** Streak ovaries

☐ **D** Cubitus valgus

☐ **E** Webbed neck

2 Select TWO of the following. Pertussis immunisation is contraindicated in a child

☐ **A** with atopic eczema

☐ **B** who develops fever of 40 °C within 36 hours of the first dose of the triple vaccine

☐ **C** whose maternal uncle is an epileptic

☐ **D** who develops a severe local reaction at the site where the first dose of the triple vaccine was administered

☐ **E** who had hypocalcaemic fits in the neonatal period

3 Which TWO of the following are true of infectious hepatitis?

☐ **A** Hepatitis C is food/water-borne

☐ **B** Patients are maximally infectious prior to the onset of jaundice

☐ **C** Vaccine to hepatitis B may reduce the incidence of hepatoma

☐ **D** Alkaline phosphatase is rarely more than double the upper limit of the reference range

☐ **E** Hepatitis D is now the commonest blood-borne hepatitis in the UK

4   Which THREE of the following are features of glandular fever?

☐ **A**   Abnormal liver function tests

☐ **B**   Rash

☐ **C**   Illness lasts about five days

☐ **D**   Monospot test is invariably positive

☐ **E**   Gross cervical lymphadenopathy

5   Which TWO of the following statements about normal iron metabolism are true?

☐ **A**   The normal daily requirement for adults is 1–2 mg

☐ **B**   Haemoglobin accounts for about 25% of total body iron

☐ **C**   There is no physiological route for iron excretion

☐ **D**   Iron is more readily absorbed from vegetables than from meat

6   Pneumococcal immunisation should be given to which TWO groups of patients?

☐ **A**   Patients who are HIV-positive

☐ **B**   Patients who are heterozygous for Hb S

☐ **C**   Patients who have had a splenectomy

☐ **D**   Every five years where indicated

☐ **E**   Prior to travel to countries with high rates of penicillin-resistant pneumococci

7 **Which THREE conditions increase patients' susceptibility to pneumococcal infections?**

- [ ] **A** Hypothyroidism
- [ ] **B** Post-splenectomy
- [ ] **C** Melanoma
- [ ] **D** Multiple myeloma
- [ ] **E** Anaemia
- [ ] **F** Sickle cell disease

SINGLE BEST ANSWER QUESTIONS

1   Select the statement which is NOT true of measles

☐   **A**   Accounts for 15% of deaths from all causes in children under five in developed countries

☐   **B**   May cause recurrent pneumothoraces

☐   **C**   May cause corneal ulceration

☐   **D**   Is more dangerous in overcrowded households

☐   **E**   Establishes lifelong immunity after natural infection

2   Which of the following does NOT result in a depressed immune response?

☐   **A**   Obesity

☐   **B**   Antibiotic treatment

☐   **C**   Renal failure

☐   **D**   Old age

☐   **E**   Infection

3   Which of the following is NOT associated with red blood cell macrocytosis?

☐   **A**   Coeliac disease

☐   **B**   Ulcerative colitis

☐   **C**   Alcoholism

☐   **D**   Aplastic anaemia

4 **Deficiencies of the following food substances are linked with which ONE of the associated haematological conditions?**

☐ **A** Iron and megaloblastic anaemia

☐ **B** Cobalamin and haemolytic anaemia

☐ **C** Folic acid and microcytic anaemia

☐ **D** Vitamin C and microcytic anaemia

5 **Which of the following statements is NOT true about sickle cell anaemia?**

☐ **A** Folate supplements may prevent aplastic crises

☐ **B** Serum iron is low

☐ **C** Aseptic femoral head necrosis may occur

☐ **D** Priapism is a recognised complication

☐ **E** Pneumococcal immunisation is advised

☐ **F** Recurrent haematuria may occur

6 **Which ONE of the following is NOT a complication of rheumatoid disease?**

☐ **A** Finger clubbing

☐ **B** Baker's synovial cysts

☐ **C** Pleural effusion

☐ **D** Leg ulcers

☐ **E** Pernicious anaemia

PHOTO QUESTION

THEME: INFECTION

For each image, select the most appropriate treatment.

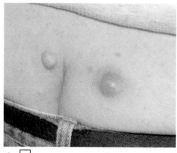

1 ☐

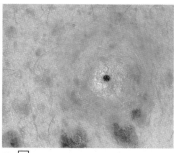

2 ☐

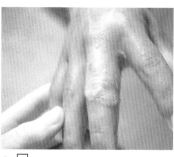

3 ☐

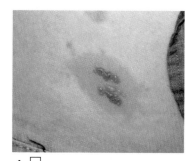

4 ☐

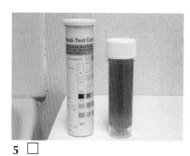

5 ☐

A   Trimethoprim.

B   Aciclovir.

C   Miconazole.

D   Incision and curettage.

E   Flucloxacillin.

PAEDIATRICS

EXTENDED MATCHING QUESTIONS

THEME: COMMON DEVELOPMENTAL MILESTONES

A 3 months

B 6 months

C 9 months

D 12 months

E 18 months

For each of the descriptions, select the single most likely age. Each option may be used once, more than once, or not at all.

1 Says two to three words with meaning. ☐

2 Sits unsupported and may crawl on abdomen. ☐

3 Manages a spoon. ☐

4 Builds a three- to four-cube tower. ☐

5 Sits supported. ☐

6 Holds object placed in hand. ☐

7 Walks with one hand held. ☐

THEME: ABDOMINAL PAIN IN CHILDREN

A   Inguinal hernia

B   Urinary tract infection

C   Sickle cell disease

D   Intussusception

E   Acute porphyria

F   Diabetic ketoacidosis

G   Henoch-Schönlein purpura

H   Appendicitis

I   Abdominal migraine

J   Testicular torsion

K   Lead poisoning

L   Mesenteric adenitis

From the list of descriptions below, select the most likely diagnosis from the list above. Each option may be used once, more than once, or not at all.

8   Usually associated with a rash and joint swelling, often with haematuria. ☐

9   Is characterised by periodic bouts of screaming, drawing up of the legs and pallor, with blood-stained mucus passed in nappies. ☐

10   Should be considered in a child with abdominal pain and dysuria, with normal urine. ☐

11   May cause referred pain to the abdomen in 25% of cases. ☐

12   May be associated with preceding upper respiratory tract symptoms. ☐

MULTIPLE BEST ANSWER QUESTIONS

1   Select THREE risk factors for sudden infant death syndrome

☐ **A**   Female sex

☐ **B**   Supine sleeping position

☐ **C**   Young maternal age

☐ **D**   Low parity

☐ **E**   Winter months

☐ **F**   Respiratory symptoms over the previous few days

2   Select THREE statements about breast-feeding

☐ **A**   Is protective against gastrointestinal infections

☐ **B**   Reduces the risk of insulin-dependent diabetes

☐ **C**   Is protective against respiratory diseases

☐ **D**   Increases the risk of maternal breast cancer

☐ **E**   Increases the likelihood of childhood obesity

3   Select THREE factors that are less common in breast-fed babies

☐ **A**   Non-accidental injury

☐ **B**   Coeliac disease

☐ **C**   Eczema

☐ **D**   Urinary tract infections

☐ **E**   Cot death

4 Select THREE common features of Down's syndrome

☐ **A** Speckled iris (Brushfield's spots)

☐ **B** Normal IQ

☐ **C** Loose skin on the nape of the neck

☐ **D** Protruding tongue

☐ **E** Spasticity

5 Select THREE statements regarding congenital dislocation of the hip

☐ **A** It is more common in boys than in girls

☐ **B** In carrying out Ortolani's test the hips should be abducted to 70°

☐ **C** Is a cause of delayed walking

☐ **D** Treatment is most effective in infants

☐ **E** When picked up late, requires an open reduction operation

6 People with Down's syndrome are particularly prone to which TWO conditions?

☐ **A** Diabetes insipidus

☐ **B** Hypothyroidism

☐ **C** Hyperparathyroidism

☐ **D** Alzheimer's disease

☐ **E** Addison's disease

7 Select TWO of the following statements about nocturnal enuresis

- ☐ **A** Most children with nocturnal enuresis are reliably dry during the day

- ☐ **B** By the age of 10 years only about 1% of children suffer nocturnal enuresis

- ☐ **C** First-born children are more prone to nocturnal enuresis than later children

- ☐ **D** Urodynamic studies can often help diagnose the cause of nocturnal enuresis

- ☐ **E** Tricyclic drugs are effective by reason of their anticholinergic and antidepressant effects

8 At the age of 8 months, a baby can be expected to do which TWO of the following?

- ☐ **A** Roll over from front to back

- ☐ **B** Pick up a small bead between thumb and finger

- ☐ **C** Sit up with a straight back

- ☐ **D** Say up to five words clearly

- ☐ **E** Feed himself or herself with a spoon

SINGLE BEST ANSWER QUESTIONS

1 In congenital dislocation of the hip which of the following is true?

☐ **A** The incidence is 2–3 per 100 births in the UK

☐ **B** The rate of surgical intervention has changed with screening

☐ **C** Splinting carries a risk of avascular necrosis of the femoral head

2 Which of the following statements is NOT true about congenital dislocation of the hip?

☐ **A** It is more common in males

☐ **B** Ninety per cent of dislocatable hips will stabilise in the first two months of life

☐ **C** It is rare in black Afro-Caribbean people

☐ **D** It is best diagnosed using ultrasound rather than X-rays

☐ **E** The risk is increased with a positive family history

3 Which of the following is true of puberty?

☐ **A** In normal girls the pubertal growth spurt precedes the menarche

☐ **B** The first sign of puberty in the male is development of pubic hair

☐ **C** Precocious puberty is more likely to have a sinister underlying cause in a girl than in a boy

☐ **D** Delayed pubertal development is most commonly due to a structural defect causing gonadotrophin deficiency

☐ **E** Menarche is a late event in puberty

PHOTO QUESTION

THEME: LOWER LIMBS

For each image, select the case description which is most likely to correspond to the history.

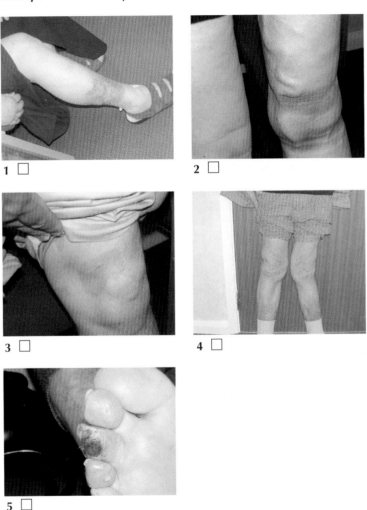

1 ☐

2 ☐

3 ☐

4 ☐

5 ☐

A An autosomal dominant condition associated with acoustic neuromas.

B Conservative treatment may avoid long term complications.

C Often pain free on waking, discomfort worsens towards the end of the day.

D Associated with diabetes.

E Associated with atrial fibrillation.

PHARMACO-THERAPEUTICS

EXTENDED MATCHING QUESTIONS

THEME: COMPLEMENTARY MEDICINE

A Angus castus

B Butterbur

C Feverfew

D Garlic

E Ginger

F Ginkgo

G St John's wort

H Saw palmetto

Choose one of the above options for each of the following statements.
Each option may be used once, more than once, or not at all.

1 Used in the treatment of benign prostatic hypertrophy. ☐

2 Used in pre-menstrual syndrome. ☐

3 Popularly used in depression. ☐

4 Used in memory loss and dementia, but should be avoided in people taking aspirin and warfarin. ☐

5 Has numerous drug interactions, and reduces the level of the oral contraceptive pill. ☐

6 Used in the treatment of hayfever. ☐

THEME: SIMILAR-SOUNDING DRUGS

A Lansoprazole

B Lofepramine

C Loperamide

D Loprazolam

E Loratadine

F Lorazepam

For each description below, select the single most likely drug from the above options. Each option may be used once, more than once, or not at all.

7 An antihistamine. ☐

8 Can cause abdominal cramps and is used as an adjunct to other treatment in diarrhoea. ☐

9 A proton pump inhibitor. ☐

10 A hypnotic. ☐

11 An anxiolytic and can be used in the treatment of status epilepticus. ☐

12 Used in the symptomatic treatment of urticaria. ☐

13 Used in the treatment of duodenal ulcers. ☐

14 An antidepressant. ☐

THEME: SIDE-EFFECTS OF DYSPEPSIA TREATMENT

A Aluminium salts

B H$_2$-receptor antagonists

C Magnesium salts

D Metoclopramide

E Misoprostol

F Omeprazole

For each side-effect, select the single most likely dyspepsia treatment. Each option may be used once, more than once, or not at all.

15 Can cause inter-menstrual bleeding. ☐

16 Can be associated with post-menopausal bleeding. ☐

17 Often causes diarrhoea. ☐

18 Can cause severe skin reactions and photosensitivity. ☐

19 Frequently causes constipation. ☐

20 Is associated with dystonic reactions. ☐

21 Can cause galactorrhoea. ☐

22 Can cause confusion, which is reversible on stopping the medication. ☐

THEME: ANTI-INFECTIVE DRUG SIDE-EFFECTS

A Aciclovir

B Azithromycin

C Ciprofloxacin

D Doxycycline

E Metronidazole

F Rifampicin

G Terbinafine

H Zanamivir

For each side-effect described, select the drug associated with it. Each option may be used once, more than once, or not at all.

23 Acute renal failure. ☐

24 Bronchospasm. ☐

25 Photosensitivity. ☐

26 Discoloration of body secretions. ☐

27 Tendon damage. ☐

28 Disulfiram-like reaction. ☐

MULTIPLE BEST ANSWER QUESTIONS

1   Which TWO of the following drugs should be avoided in renal failure?

☐ **A**   Ampicillin

☐ **B**   Oxytetracycline

☐ **C**   Aluminium hydroxide

☐ **D**   Ferrous sulphate

☐ **E**   Nitrofurantoin

2   Choose TWO of the following statements. Benzodiazepine anxiolytics

☐ **A**   have no active metabolites

☐ **B**   differ significantly in their duration of action

☐ **C**   differ significantly in their sedative effect relative to anxiolytic activity

☐ **D**   increase body sway

3   Select TWO statements about cannabis

☐ **A**   It is usually smoked but can be ingested or injected intravenously

☐ **B**   Usually causes bradycardia

☐ **C**   Injections produce severe constipation

☐ **D**   Use over many years may impair academic performance, but this is reversible on cessation of use

☐ **E**   Smoke may be carcinogenic

4 **Aspirin potentiates the therapeutic action of which TWO drugs?**

☐ **A** Warfarin

☐ **B** Probenecid

☐ **C** Indometacin

☐ **D** Diazepam

☐ **E** Tetracyclines

5 **Which THREE of the following drugs should be avoided or used with caution in renal failure?**

☐ **A** Aspirin

☐ **B** Ampicillin

☐ **C** Glibenclamide

☐ **D** Somatropin

☐ **E** Atorvastatin

6 **Which TWO of the following are associated with cannabis abuse?**

☐ **A** Irreversible reduction in academic performance

☐ **B** Persistent bradycardia

☐ **C** Hypotension

☐ **D** Hypertension

☐ **E** Status epilepticus

7 **Choose THREE recognised side-effects of benzodiazepines from the following list**

☐ **A** Confusion

☐ **B** Impaired driving skills

☐ **C** Potentiation of the effects of alcohol

☐ **D** Aplastic anaemia

☐ **E** Convulsions

8 **Which THREE of the following drugs are safe to use in combination with warfarin?**

☐ **A** Ranitidine

☐ **B** Co-trimoxazole

☐ **C** Carbamazepine

☐ **D** Ibuprofen

☐ **E** Salbutamol

9 **There is reduced effectiveness of the combined oral contraceptive pill following interaction with which THREE of the following?**

☐ **A** Rifamycins

☐ **B** Carbamazepine

☐ **C** Warfarin

☐ **D** Lisinopril

☐ **E** Griseofulvin

10 **Which TWO of the following side-effects are linked with non-steroidal anti-inflammatory drugs?**

☐ **A** Hypokalaemia

☐ **B** Polycythaemia

☐ **C** Neutrophilia

☐ **D** Thrombocytopenia

☐ **E** Hypocalcaemia

SINGLE BEST ANSWER QUESTIONS

1 Which ONE of the following drugs is contraindicated in breast-feeding?

☐ **A** Warfarin

☐ **B** Senna

☐ **C** Digoxin

☐ **D** Paracetamol

☐ **E** Cimetidine

2 Which ONE of these statements about zanamivir (Relenza®) is NOT correct?

☐ **A** Inhibits viral replication

☐ **B** Does not work with influenza B infections

☐ **C** Is given as a nasal spray or dry powder inhaler

☐ **D** Is of particular benefit when symptoms have been present for less than 30 hours

☐ **E** May exacerbate asthma

☐ **F** Enables patients to return to work more quickly

3 Which ONE of these statements about St John's wort is NOT true?

☐ **A** Is no more effective than placebo in depression

☐ **B** Can induce liver enzymes

☐ **C** Is used widely in the UK

☐ **D** Interacts with digoxin

☐ **E** Interacts with warfarin

4   Which ONE of the following is NOT a toxic effect of digoxin therapy?

☐ **A**   Abdominal pain

☐ **B**   Visual disturbance

☐ **C**   T wave inversion

☐ **D**   Prolonged PR interval

☐ **E**   Anorexia

5   Which ONE of the following statements is NOT true about warfarin?

☐ **A**   Reduces vitamin-K-dependent clotting factors

☐ **B**   Reacts with ampicillin to increase anticoagulant effect

☐ **C**   Appears in breast milk in quantities too small to affect the baby

☐ **D**   Has an increased anticoagulant effect with griseofulvin therapy

6   Which ONE of the following is true about glibenclamide?

☐ **A**   It has a shorter half-life than chlorpropamide

☐ **B**   It does not cross the placenta

☐ **C**   It is safe in renal impairment

☐ **D**   It is safe to use in the elderly

SUMMARY COMPLETION QUESTION

THEME: OVER-THE-COUNTER REMEDIES

Read the extract from the paper below which describes lay beliefs about OTC cough and cold remedies, then read the summary below and choose appropriate responses for each challenge from the list below.

Remedy or cure? Lay beliefs about over-the-counter medicines for coughs and colds. Johnson and Helman *British Journal of General Practice* 2004;54:98–102

Abstract

Aim To examine lay beliefs about over-the-counter medicines for coughs and colds. To explore whether the distinction between symptom relief and cure has the same relevance to lay people as it does to medical professionals.

Design of study Small pilot study using qualitative techniques.

Setting Variety sample of 11 patients attending the National Health Service walk-in centre, Birmingham, England.

The main researcher has gathered anecdotal evidence, over 20 years' work as a general practitioner (GP), that her patients' beliefs about the effects of over-the-counter medicines often diverged from conventional medical opinion. This study was designed to explore lay beliefs about these medicines in more depth.

Method

A GP acted as an observer during consultations with nurses at a National Health Service (NHS) walk-in centre in Birmingham, which is in the basement of the main branch of 'Boots The Chemists' pharmacy. She was introduced as 'a colleague', although some patients recognised that she was a doctor. She approached 20 patients (chosen as a heterogeneous sample of ages, ethnic groups and occupations) after their consultations. Eleven of these agreed to be interviewed in depth; their ages ranged from 21 to 77 years, and six of them were women. The information sheet explained that participants' opinions were being sought about over-the-counter medicines, and written consent was obtained. Ethical approval was obtained from South Birmingham Local Research Ethics Committee.

Face-to-face interviews were conducted using a semi-structured questionnaire. The participants were asked about the medicines that they normally used for coughs and colds, and their views about the effectiveness of these medicines. Both open-ended and more direct questions were used, to allow them to explain their own perspective. In addition, they were invited to comment on several fictional case histories involving the use of over-the-counter medicines to treat coughs and colds. During the interviews, the interviewer was careful not to express her own opinion, or to describe any 'official' views about these medicines. Answers to the questionnaire were taken in note form and transcribed verbatim.

Participants were then asked to take part in a pile-sorting exercise, designed to further test their understanding about the distinction between symptom relief and 'cure'. This research technique involved giving them, in random order, cards bearing the names of different medicines used for coughs and colds, and asking them to put the cards on one of three piles labelled 'This will shorten a cough or cold', 'This will relieve coughs and colds only for a few hours' and 'Don't know'. The names of the over-the-counter medicines on the cards are given in Box 1.

Cross-checking of the data was carried out to identify any inconsistencies between the responses to the questionnaire, case vignettes and pile-sorting. The answers were analysed in order to discover common themes, which were compared with existing themes identified in the recent anthropological literature.

Summary

The objective of this study is to examine the beliefs of the general public regarding over-the-counter remedies, and to explore the understanding of the difference between symptom relief and cure. It is not clear what the application of this knowledge will be: are the researchers attempting to analyse health seeking behaviour when challenged by coughs or colds, or are they attempting to understand the economics of the cough remedy market? This study does not aim to confirm or refute____**(1)**____, rather it aims to collect____**(2)**____ data on beliefs.

The study setting was an NHS walk-in centre, with the observer sitting in on consultations and then approaching a selection of patients after their consultation. Although this was a____**(3)**____ study, this approach has significant implications when the results are considered. Such studies are used to trial a line of enquiry to see if a larger more definitive study is feasible. Their aim is not statistically significant results, and indeed are almost by definition ____**(4)**____ to generate such results, but the methodology must be sound to allow____**(5)**____to larger projects.

The authors have clearly made little allowance for____**(6)**____ in planning their study. The error is in the setting. Members of the public who present to an NHS walk-in centre are probably not representative of the general public, and may well have health beliefs which differ from patients presenting at a GP surgery. This setting is unlikely to generate a ____**(7)**____ cross-section of the public. Furthermore the NHS walk-in centre is located in the basement of a chemist; hence it is unlikely to be frequented by people who don't believe in the effectiveness of over-the-counter remedies. A further source of selection bias lies in the recruitment of participants. The observer sitting in on consultations, and then approaching patients____**(8)**____ after witnessing first hand their health beliefs at work, is highly likely to bias selection in favour of certain beliefs. No mention is made of the recruitment process – were all patients approached or just a select few? If a select few, how were they selected? What were the initial presentations of the participants? Were they presenting with specific cough and cold queries or selected from a diverse group? Again, this may bias the results.

The secondary aim of the study was to determine if lay beliefs in the distinction between symptom relief and cure differ from those of the medical profession, but does it matter? Coughs and colds are benign, self-limiting conditions where the distinction is academic, since symptom relief for a few days will see the patient almost always recover. This group of patients have chosen to self-medicate or use alternatives rather than present to their GP, and since we have no effective cure for the common cold, there seems little benefit in challenging mistaken beliefs in the curing abilities of over-the-counter remedies. Perhaps education regarding the _____(9)_____ of common illnesses should be aimed at pharmacists and their staff, to reassure patients when selling them their largely ineffective cough remedies and prevent them presenting unnecessarily to their GP. The author concludes the introduction with the information that the main researcher has spent 20 years gathering anecdotal evidence about this subject. Flawed _____(10)_____ and failure to minimise bias mean that this study adds little more than further anecdote.

Options

A   Bias

B   Controls

C   Underpowered

D   Sample size

E   Qualitative

F   Causation

G   Post hoc

H   Unable

I   Working hypotheses

J   Extrapolation

K   Ad hoc

L   Pilot

M   Natural history

N   Selection

O   Representative

P   Quantitative

Q   Methodology

R   Random

S   Argument

PSYCHIATRY/NEUROLOGY

EXTENDED MATCHING QUESTIONS

THEME: SECTIONS OF THE MENTAL HEALTH ACT

A   Section 2

B   Section 3

C   Section 4

D   Section 5

E   Section 7

For each of the statements, select the single most likely section. Each of the options may be used once, more than once, or not at all.

1 Is suitable to use when considering guardianship ☐

2 Is most suitable for a patient with a recurrence of a mental illness associated with non-compliance with treatment ☐

3 Is used in an emergency to bring someone into hospital for a full assessment of the mental state ☐

4 Is used in an emergency to keep someone in hospital pending a further assessment ☐

5 Is normally used to admit a patient to hospital for a full assessment of the mental state ☐

THEME: HEADACHES

A   Cluster headache

B   Migraine

C   Referred from neck

D   Tension headache

For each of the descriptions, select the most likely type of headache. Each option may be used once, more than once, or not at all.

6 The patient will commonly show pallor. ☐

7 The pain is typically diffuse or bilateral. ☐

8 The pain is described as a 'weight on the top of the head' or as a 'band'. ☐

9 The patient often experiences flushing. ☐

10 The patient often complains of a watery eye. ☐

THEME: DISC LESIONS

A   At L2–L3 level

B   At L5–S1 level

C   Central disc prolapse

For each of the descriptions, select the most likely level of disc lesion. Each option may be used once, more than once, or not at all.

11 There will characteristically be loss of ankle reflex. ☐

12 There will usually be loss of bladder function. ☐

13 The femoral stretch test will be positive. ☐

THEME: QUESTIONNAIRES

A CAGE

B CRATE

C EAT

D MAST

E SCOFF

For each of the descriptions, select the single most likely questionnaire. Each option may be used once, more than once, or not at all.

14 This is a questionnaire to identify people with alcohol problems, who commonly score over 6 with these questions. ☐

15 This looks at people with eating disorders. ☐

16 This detects people with alcohol problems, who will probably score between 2 and 4. ☐

17 This questionnaire asks, among other questions, whether the person has been arrested for drunken driving. ☐

THEME: HEADACHE

A   Chronic daily headache

B   Cluster headache

C   Coital cephalgia

D   Migraine with aura

E   Migraine without aura

F   Sinusitis

G   Subarachnoid haemorrhage

H   Temporal arteritis

I   Tension headache

J   Trigeminal neuralgia

For each of the descriptions listed below, select the single most appropriate answer. Each answer may be used once, more than once, or not at all.

18 May occur every day, be continuous and worsen through the day; rarely disturbs sleep; patients can usually work through them; often band-like with associated neck and shoulder stiffness. ☐

19 Seen mostly in men – a sudden onset of severe pain; may be confused with subarachnoid haemorrhage. ☐

20 Characterised by bouts of daily pain occurring for weeks or months at a time, always unilateral and centred on the eye or cheek, often with lacrimation. ☐

21 Causes recurrent severe unilateral headache with nausea and photophobia, often preceded by a prodromal phase. ☐

22 May rapidly cause blindness if untreated. ☐

23 Is a contraindication to the combined contraceptive pill. ☐

THEME: PSYCHIATRIC COMPLAINTS

A Anxiety disorder

B Bipolar disorder

C Borderline personality disorder

D Conversion disorder

E Dementia

F Drug-induced psychosis

G Obsessive-compulsive personality disorder

H Post-traumatic stress disorder

I Schizoid personality disorder

J Schizophrenia

For each clinical scenario described below, select the single most likely diagnosis from the list above. Each answer may be used once, more than once, or not at all.

24 A 77-year-old man complains that he cannot play bridge any more due to his inability to memorise hands. Despite his legendary recall of people having long since passed away, his wife says they frequently argue about his failure to remember what they need from the shops. ☐

25 A 44-year-old woman is brought in by her estranged partner, having awoken that morning unable to speak. He is very concerned but she is able to put a brave face on things. She can cough and swallow and ENT examination is normal. ☐

26 Mrs Smith, a 33-year-old woman, was involved in a minor road traffic accident last year. She frequently suffers a dry mouth, difficulty breathing and palpitations. She has trouble sleeping and her memory has deteriorated. ☐

27 A 22-year-old man asks for a sick note to cover his absence from community service last week. He has been in prison for joyriding and theft, and on occasions has threatened suicide. The receptionists in the past have complained about his aggressive and intimidating behaviour. ☐

28 You are called by a neighbour to visit a 67-year-old woman with a previous history of depression. He found her dancing in the garden naked at 3 am last night. She has not slept for days and is bizarrely dressed. She denies there is a problem – she feels fantastic. ☐

29 Since starting university Tom has become interested in the paranormal, is increasingly dishevelled and has been seen talking to himself. His mother says he recently covered the TV screen with paper. He is suspicious and his speech seems to flit from one unrelated theme to another. ☐

THEME: MIGRAINE

A Aspirin

B Avoidance of trigger factors

C Co-codamol

D Emergency medical referral

E Ergotamine

F IM pethidine

G PR diclofenac

H Referral to Neurology Outpatients

I Sumatriptan

For each of the descriptions below, select the most appropriate option from the list above. Each option may be used once, more than once, or not at all.

30 First-line treatment. ☐

31 Should be considered as a prophylactic measure in all patients. ☐

32 Should be considered if first-line treatment fails to abort an attack. ☐

33 For regular severe attacks, unresponsive to simple remedies. Should be taken as soon as possible after an attack starts. ☐

34 Is a contraindication to combined oral contraceptive use. ☐

35 Should be considered for sudden-onset severe headaches with atypical features. ☐

THEME: HEADACHES

A Alcoholism

B Brain tumour

C Carbon monoxide poisoning

D Cervical spondylosis

E Depression

F Migraine

G Temporal arteritis

H Tension headache

Select the most likely diagnosis as the cause of the headache. Each option may be used once, more than once, or not at all.

36 A 70-year-old man with a 3-week history of left-sided headache and one day of blurring vision.

37 A 20-year-old girl recently moved in with her boyfriend, complaining of recent onset of frequent headaches, usually on the right side, accompanied by nausea.

38 A 55-year-old male General Practitioner with morning headaches over the last six months, accompanied by strange avoidance behaviour, vomiting and weight loss.

39 A 35-year-old lady with polyarthralgia, muscle pains, palpitations and lethargy.

40 A 25-year-old who has just moved into your area into a bedsit, who calls you out with headache, vomiting and says she is unable to get out of bed, but who looks remarkably well in terms of 'colour'.

THEME: MRC SCALE FOR MUSCLE POWER

A 0

B ½

C 1

D 2

E 3

F 4

G 4½

H 5

For each of the descriptions, select the most likely number. Each of the options may be used once, more than once, or not at all.

41 Movement overcomes gravity plus added resistance. ☐

42 No movement of the joint, but visible muscle contraction. ☐

43 Normal power. ☐

THEME: NERVE ROOT LESIONS

A C4

B C5

C C6

D C6/7

E L3/4

F L5/S1

G S1/S2

For each of the clinical scenarios, select the single most appropriate nerve root lesion. Each option may be used once, more than once, or not at all.

44 Absent ankle reflex and poor foot plantarflexion, but knee flexion intact. ☐

45 Absent biceps reflex and poor shoulder abduction. ☐

46 Absent supinator reflex and poor elbow flexion, but triceps reflex present. ☐

47 Absent knee reflex and poor knee extension and foot dorsiflexion. ☐

MULTIPLE BEST ANSWER QUESTIONS

1   **Which two of the following are diagnostic criteria for bulimia nervosa?**

☐   **A**   Frequent binges

☐   **B**   Little concern about shape

☐   **C**   Little concern about weight

☐   **D**   Low weight

☐   **E**   Behaviour such as vomiting or fasting to prevent weight gain

2   **In a 70-year-old man with tremor of the upper limbs, essential tremor rather than Parkinson's disease is more likely to be the cause in which TWO of the following?**

☐   **A**   The tremor is worst at rest

☐   **B**   The tremor is relieved with alcohol

☐   **C**   The tremor is exacerbated by anxiety

☐   **D**   The tremor is predominantly postural

☐   **E**   There is rigidity

3   **Select FOUR important risk factors for suicide**

☐   **A**   Recent self-harm

☐   **B**   Female

☐   **C**   Married

☐   **D**   Unemployed

☐   **E**   Severity of depression

☐   **F**   Active plans

☐   **G**   Passive thoughts about being harmed

4 Select THREE factors which predispose to major depression

☐ **A** A professional background

☐ **B** A first-degree relative with major depression

☐ **C** The presence of more than three children in the house

☐ **D** Employment in the same company for more than 10 years

☐ **E** Loss of a parent before 11 years of age

5 Select TWO of the following statements regarding compensation neurosis

☐ **A** It has a recognised association with major rather than minor accidents

☐ **B** It occurs particularly after head injuries sustained at work

☐ **C** Settlement of a compensation claim is followed by improvement in patients with severe symptoms

☐ **D** Malingering accounts for at least 30% of cases

☐ **E** Irritability is a recognised feature

6 Select THREE statements about agoraphobia

☐ **A** Usually starts before puberty

☐ **B** Occurs more often in women than in men

☐ **C** Can be effectively treated by systematic desensitisation

☐ **D** Becomes worse during periods of depression

☐ **E** Can usually be traced back to traumatic events in childhood

7   Select THREE of the following statements concerning grief reaction

- ☐ **A** Is typically self-limiting
- ☐ **B** Characteristically includes denial
- ☐ **C** Is best treated with tricyclic antidepressants
- ☐ **D** Typically includes suicidal ideas
- ☐ **E** Is a form of psychosis

8   Select TWO of the following statements about anxiety states

- ☐ **A** Chest pain may be a presenting symptom
- ☐ **B** May present with persistent memory impairment
- ☐ **C** Difficulty in exhaling is common
- ☐ **D** Low mood and early morning wakening are invariably present
- ☐ **E** Sweating is quite common

9   Select TWO of the following about obsessive-compulsive disorder

- ☐ **A** Obsessional thoughts are recognised by patients as being their own
- ☐ **B** Women are more commonly affected than men
- ☐ **C** Obsessional thoughts are usually pleasant in nature
- ☐ **D** Depression is unusual
- ☐ **E** Two-thirds of cases have improved at the end of one year

10 Select THREE Schneiderian first-rank symptoms of schizophrenia

- ☐ **A** Thought insertion
- ☐ **B** Visual hallucinations
- ☐ **C** Suicidal ideas
- ☐ **D** Passivity phenomena
- ☐ **E** Thought broadcast

11 **Select THREE of the following. An acute confusional state is**

☐ **A** Often responsive to tricyclic antidepressant drug therapy

☐ **B** A characteristic feature of myxoedema

☐ **C** Characterised by loss of memory for recent events

☐ **D** Typically reversible

☐ **E** More common with pre-existing brain disease

12 **Select THREE characteristic features of hypomania**

☐ **A** Flight of ideas

☐ **B** Thought insertion

☐ **C** Sexual promiscuity

☐ **D** Delusions of bodily illness

☐ **E** Sleep disturbance

13 **Select THREE typical features of alcohol withdrawal**

☐ **A** Dehydration

☐ **B** Visual hallucinations

☐ **C** Passivity feelings

☐ **D** Tremor

☐ **E** Confabulation

14 **Select TWO features of hysteria**

☐ **A** The physical symptom is produced deliberately

☐ **B** It may be associated with a depressive illness

☐ **C** It is associated with 'la belle indifference'

☐ **D** It characteristically occurs for the first time in middle age

☐ **E** The physical symptoms and signs closely resemble those of organic disease

15 Select FOUR of the following statements about suicide

☐ **A** Two-thirds of these who die by suicide have told someone of their intention

☐ **B** Asking about suicidal intent will increase the risk of suicide

☐ **C** Patients with chronic physical illness are at decreased risk

☐ **D** It is associated with alcohol abuse

☐ **E** It is most common in young women

☐ **F** Patients recently bereaved are at increased risk

☐ **G** Unemployed patients are at more risk than those in stressful jobs

16 Select TWO good prognostic signs in schizophrenia

☐ **A** Early onset

☐ **B** Depressive features

☐ **C** Echolalia

☐ **D** Preservation of affect

☐ **E** Visual hallucinations

17 Select TWO of the following statements about multiple sclerosis

☐ **A** Has a higher prevalence in tropical zones than in temperate zones

☐ **B** Presents as a single symptom in most patients

☐ **C** May present with diplopia due to optic nerve involvement

☐ **D** Does not cause progressive disability in up to one-third of patients

☐ **E** Very rarely causes sensory disturbance of the limbs

18 **Select THREE symptoms which are commonly associated with Bell's palsy**

☐ **A** Dry eye

☐ **B** Hyperacusis

☐ **C** Dry mouth

☐ **D** Loss of taste

☐ **E** Postauricular pain

19 **Select THREE of the following statements relating to the supply of the leg**

☐ **A** Spasticity in a patient with hemiplegia is most pronounced in the extensor muscles

☐ **B** Weakness in a patient with hemiplegia is most pronounced in the flexor muscles

☐ **C** Sensory loss affecting skin over the lateral aspect of the lower leg may be due to a femoral nerve palsy

☐ **D** Weakness of knee extension may be due to a sciatic nerve palsy

☐ **E** Foot drop may be due to a common peroneal nerve palsy

20 **Select TWO statements about multiple sclerosis**

☐ **A** Onset after the age of 40 years indicates a better prognosis

☐ **B** Magnetic resonance imaging may be useful in confirming the diagnosis

☐ **C** Initial presentation with motor symptoms indicates a better prognosis

☐ **D** A homonymous hemianopia is a common feature

☐ **E** Red–green colour vision may be impaired

21 Select TWO comments about stroke

☐ **A** The third most common cause of death in the UK

☐ **B** More commonly caused by infarction than haemorrhage

☐ **C** More common among people from higher socioeconomic classes

☐ **D** More likely to be fatal if caused by infarction than haemorrhage

☐ **E** Linked to raised systolic blood pressure but not diastolic

SINGLE BEST ANSWER QUESTIONS

1   Which ONE of the following is true of Alzheimer's disease?

☐   **A**   Behavioural disturbance is an early clinical manifestation

☐   **B**   Extensor plantar responses and myoclonus are early clinical features

☐   **C**   The EEG is usually normal

☐   **D**   It is associated with a predominantly frontal cortical distribution of pathology

☐   **E**   It is usually familial

☐   **F**   It is the commonest cause of dementia

2   In the differential diagnosis of dementia which ONE of the following is true?

☐   **A**   A multi-infarct aetiology is more common than the Alzheimer's type

☐   **B**   A CT scan will reliably distinguish between Alzheimer's and multi-infarct dementia

☐   **C**   In Alzheimer's disease a gait disorder is seen at an early stage

☐   **D**   In Creutzfeldt-Jakob disease an EEG may be characteristic

3   Which ONE of the following is true with regard to alcohol?

☐   **A**   Consumption of 7–21 units per month is associated with the lowest mortality

☐   **B**   Problems can almost all be identified by a raised mean cell volume (MCV) and raised gamma-GT

☐   **C**   Problems may be picked up by the use of a CAGE questionnaire, with only 25% of those with problems scoring 2 or more

4   Which ONE of the following factors does not indicate an increased risk of suicide in a depressed patient?

- ☐ **A**   A direct statement of intent to commit suicide
- ☐ **B**   Hopelessness
- ☐ **C**   Pressure of serious physical illness
- ☐ **D**   Living alone
- ☐ **E**   Presence of paranoid delusions

5   Which ONE of the following is NOT true of chronic fatigue syndrome?

- ☐ **A**   Previous psychiatric illness is a recognised risk factor
- ☐ **B**   A mild rise in creatine phosphokinase is commonly detected
- ☐ **C**   Persistent viral antigen is detected in a minority of patients
- ☐ **D**   Decreased physical activity is a risk factor for the continuation of fatigue
- ☐ **E**   The majority of affected patients fulfil psychiatric criteria for depression

6   Which ONE of the following statements regarding tricyclic antidepressants is false?

- ☐ **A**   Are contraindicated in patients with glaucoma
- ☐ **B**   May cause a dry mouth
- ☐ **C**   Are safe in patients anticoagulated with warfarin
- ☐ **D**   Are contraindicated in patients with ischaemic heart disease
- ☐ **E**   Can cause a fine tremor and inco-ordination

7 You see a 71-year-old man who eight days ago experienced an attack of shingles. He now complains of persistent pain. You make a diagnosis of post-herpetic neuralgia. Which ONE of the following is the single best treatment?

☐ **A** Aciclovir

☐ **B** Topical hydrocortisone

☐ **C** Topical capsaicin

☐ **D** Oral gabapentin

☐ **E** Epidural morphine

8 Which ONE of these structures is NOT involved in motor neurone disease?

☐ **A** Posterior horns of the spinal cord

☐ **B** Corticospinal tract

☐ **C** Corticobulbar fibres originating in the motor and pre-motor cortex

☐ **D** Nuclei of the nerves to the bulbar musculature

☐ **E** Anterior horns of the spinal cord

9 Which ONE of the following treatments may reduce the severity of relapse in multiple sclerosis?

☐ **A** Pulsed high-dose methylprednisolone

☐ **B** Adrenocortical trophic hormone (ACTH)

☐ **C** Hyperbaric oxygen

☐ **D** Azathioprine

☐ **E** Linoleic acid supplementation

10 Which ONE of the following statements about migraine is true?

- [ ] **A** Over half of all patients have their first attack before the age of 20
- [ ] **B** Over half of all patients have an aura before the headache
- [ ] **C** Frequency of attacks may vary from occasional to daily
- [ ] **D** To make the diagnosis of migraine the headache must be unilateral
- [ ] **E** Vasoconstriction of cerebral blood vessels is characteristic of migraine

11 You see a 42-year-old man with backache. Which ONE of the following symptoms may indicate potentially serious pathology and hence requires further investigation or referral if the symptoms do not resolve?

- [ ] **A** Unilateral leg pain worse than low back pain
- [ ] **B** Pain radiating to the buttocks
- [ ] **C** Perineal anaesthesia
- [ ] **D** Under 20 years or over 55 years at initial presentation
- [ ] **E** Localised neurological signs

SUMMARY COMPLETION QUESTION

THEME: COELIAC DISEASE AND SCHIZOPHRENIA

Population studies suggest that there may be a link between schizophrenia and coeliac disease. Read the extract below, and then the critique that follows. For each gap in the critique, select the most appropriate option from the list.

Coeliac disease and schizophrenia: population based case control study with linkage of Danish national registers. Eaton et al *British Medical Journal* 2004;328:438–9

Introduction

Dohan proposed that an inherited defect interacting with an environmental trigger of gluten precipitated schizophrenia in some individuals, and provided supportive epidemiological evidence. Some clinical trials and case studies showed that a cereal free diet improved remission of symptoms of schizophrenia. The most important genetic marker found in the study of coeliac disease (6p23-p22.3) is very close to the dysbindin locus, which has been implicated in schizophrenia.

Methods

The case sample comprised 7997 people older than 15 who were admitted to a Danish psychiatric facility for the first time between 1981 and 1998 with a diagnosis of schizophrenia and known maternal identity. For each case we randomly selected 25 controls from a subsample of all available controls, matched by year of birth and sex.

We searched records of the national patients' register for a history of autoimmune diseases in cases, controls, and their parents, in a manner that protected the anonymity of the participants. Denmark has few private health facilities, and treatment is free of charge, so that coverage of visits is nearly 100% complete. Diagnoses were according to the International Classification of Diseases (8th revision, 1981–94; 10th revision, 1995–8). We included coeliac disease (and closely related dermatitis herpetiformis), on the basis of prior scientific literature, and two autoimmune gastrointestinal conditions (ulcerative colitis and Crohn's disease), for which little or no scientific literature exists that implies an association with schizophrenia. We included major risk factors for schizophrenia because these might be confounders of an association with coeliac disease: socioeconomic position, urban residence, and family history of schizophrenia. Four patients, five mothers of patients, and three fathers of patients were being treated for coeliac disease before the patient entered a psychiatric facility (1.5 per 1000 population, table). In a conditional logistic regression model the relation of risk factors for schizophrenia replicated that found in the literature. The univariate relative risk for schizophrenia, given coeliac disease, was 3.2 ($P > 0.0001$), unchanged by addition of the covariates (table). The adjusted relative risks for Crohn's disease and ulcerative colitis, when using the covariates discussed above, were both 1.4 ($P > 0.08$ for Crohn's disease, and $P > 0.03$ for ulcerative colitis). When coeliac disease and four additional cases of dermatitis herpetiformis were combined in an adjusted model as described above, the relative incidence for either of the two disorders compared with neither disorder was 3.1 (95% confidence interval 1.8 to 5.2).

Comment

A history of coeliac disease is a risk factor for schizophrenia, as shown in this epidemiological study. The risk relation is strong but reflects a small proportion of cases of either disorder, since both disorders are rare.

Critique

This paper sets out to investigate the possibility of a link between schizophrenia and coeliac disease, suggested by the finding that one of the genetic markers for coeliac disease is close to one of the markers for schizophrenia. It does not attempt to prove____ **(1)**____, merely ____ **(2)**____.

Denmark is by modern standards a relatively____ **(3)**____society and the healthcare system facilitates case finding both through the near universal uptake of state healthcare and the national disease registers it maintains. This makes case finding relatively easy, providing standardisation of diagnosis when entering cases onto the register. Failure of rigorous diagnosis or coding will result in either____ **(4)**____ errors (patients misdiagnosed as cases) or____ **(5)**____errors (failure to code correctly). The first step in this study was to extract data on admissions for schizophrenia. The authors do not report whether all cases were included or whether further selection took place. This is important because schizophrenia represents a spectrum of disease and may for example include drug-induced psychosis. Furthermore this may include patients who experience an isolated psychotic episode or lifelong morbidity. Failure to control for this may influence the validity of the results.

The records of these patients and matched controls were then searched for a history of autoimmune disease. This approach relies on the coding of coeliac disease as an autoimmune disease rather than a gastro-enterological disease. The register uses diagnoses according to ICD-10, an international standard, but it is not clear who did the coding. This may be by the treating physician, which would be the most accurate method, or it may be by the register clerk, which is likely to be less accurate. Furthermore, it is unclear what the diagnostic gold standard for coeliac disease is; it may be serological, histopathological, genetic or clinical. This may further bias results. Finally, it is well established that coeliac disease is____(6)____. This could act to strengthen or weaken any association found. ____(7)____screening of cases and controls would eliminate this potential confounder.

The results are, however, impressive. The authors quote a relative risk of 3.2 for schizophrenia given coeliac disease. This could be interpreted as evidence that coeliac disease places one at a significantly increased risk of schizophrenia, however this study is not investigating aetiology. The____(8)____may be true, although unlikely, that schizophrenia causes coeliac disease. A third more likely explanation comes from the introduction. The genetic marker for coeliac disease and the dysbindin locus lie very close to each other. This will result in genetic____(9)____ and the traits will tend to be inherited together. One could choose any two genes lying close together on the same chromosome and expect them to be associated in family histories – this is, after all, the basis of genetic linkage analysis to identify gene____(10)____.

Options

A   Rare

B   Converse

C   Association

D   Location

E   Under diagnosed

F   Serological

G   Heterogeneous

H   Causation

I   Exclusion

J   Explanation

K   Homogeneous

L   Histological

M   Linkage

N   Inclusion

O   Structure

P   Pathogenesis

Q   Over diagnosed

SUMMARY COMPLETION QUESTION

THEME: GULF WAR ILLNESS

You practice in a large garrison town and have a large number of ex-military personnel registered with you. Several of them have expressed concern that they may be suffering from Gulf War illness. Your research leads you to the abstract below. Read the abstract, and the summary of the methodology below. Select from the list of options the most appropriate option for each missing word or phrase.

Gulf War illness – better, worse or just the same? A cohort study.
Hotopf *et al* British Medical Journal 2003;327:1370

Method

Participants

Our original study consisted of three groups: personnel who served in the Persian Gulf War between 1 September 1990 and 30 June 1991 (the Gulf cohort); personnel who served on UN peacekeeping duties in Bosnia between 1 April 1992 and 6 February 1997 (the Bosnia cohort); and personnel who were serving in the armed forces on 1 January 1991 but who were not deployed to the Gulf (the 'Era' cohort). We took a random sample of all Gulf veterans, with oversampling of women. Sampling of the other two cohorts was frequency matched in terms of sex, age, reservist status, officer status, service (Royal Navy, Army, or Royal Air Force), and a measure of fitness.

Of 8196 participants who responded to the first survey 503 refused permission for future contact and 449 failed to complete the relevant section of the questionnaire. We used random stratified sampling to select respondents from stage 1 into the present study. All women were selected. We stratified the sampling on the severity of fatigue at stage 1. The selection process included all male veterans with a fatigue score greater than 8 (511 Gulf, 115 Bosnia and 120 Era); for Gulf, a 50% sample of veterans with fatigue scores of 4–8 (484 veterans), along with all those in Bosnia ($n = 333$) and Era ($n = 364$) who scored in this range; and an approximately one in eight sample of veterans with fatigue scores less than 4 in order to represent asymptomatic individuals ($n = 250$ in each group).

Mailing method

We used three mailings. To trace non-responders we used the NHS central registry to obtain health authority ciphers and current addresses. We used the online electoral registry 'Cameo' to check addresses. Service pension and discharge sources supplied updated addresses. We sent the second and third mailings via commanding officers, asking for their help in disseminating the questionnaires on our behalf. Following an agreement with the War Pensions Agency, the UK Department of Social Security sent two further mailings. In order to comply with data protection regulation, we were not informed which addresses the Department of Social Security had on their records.

Questionnaire and outcomes

The questionnaire included a fatigue scale; the 12 item general health questionnaire (a screening questionnaire for common mental disorders); the SF-36 instrument for physical health and functional capacity; and a list of 50 common symptoms. We defined cases of fatigue as having a score on the fatigue scale of greater than 3 and cases of psychological distress as having a score greater than 2 on the general health questionnaire. We defined cases of 'stress reaction' from a checklist of symptoms described in previous work.

Summary

This study attempts to answer the question 'Does a history of service in the 1991 Persian Gulf conflict result in increased ill health?'. This study uses a____**(1)**____of military personnel who served in this conflict and compares them to a cohort who served in Bosnia and a control group. This is an appropriate methodology to take since the data are being collected prospectively and the study is, by definition, looking at a cohort who were exposed at the same point in time. The participants from the Gulf War cohort were____**(2)**____sampled. The characteristics of this group were then used to randomly select matched controls from the other two groups. This approach aims to minimise any major differences in the three populations which may act as confounders. Unfortunately the authors do not list the characteristics of the three groups to allow confirmation that the groups are indeed well matched.

Although the groups are well matched in terms of ages, sex, rank and fitness, they are not strictly speaking____(3)____. The cohort who served in Bosnia were involved in peacekeeping and not combat. Comparison of these groups may appear to show that service in the Gulf resulted in an increase in fatigue but in fact it may be that the underlying cause of differences in____(4)____between these groups is in fact combat. Similarly the Bosnian and Gulf war veterans are made up of potentially very different groups in terms of timescale of exposure – the Bosnian veterans are a____(5)____group who served at any time between 1992 and 1997, hence the potential lead time in which one might expect disease to develop is significantly less.

The use of self-reported fatigue as an outcome variable presents an opportunity for bias to creep in, since it is a____(6)____and potentially ill defined variable. The authors have taken steps to avoid observer bias by using a____(7)____reporting tool, and combined this with a mental health screening tool, since the outcome of fatigue is not exclusive to Gulf War illness, but could be a symptom of psychological illness and thus act as a____(8)____.

Options

A	Outcome	M	Case–control
B	Variable	N	Randomly
C	Heterogeneous	O	Selectively
D	Homogeneous	P	Comparable
E	Standardised	Q	Subjective
F	Confounder	R	Objective
G	Exclusion	S	Inclusion
H	Reporting		
I	Sampling		
J	Cohort		
K	Population		
L	Control		

REPRODUCTIVE/RENAL

EXTENDED MATCHING QUESTIONS

THEME: COMMON CANCERS

A Breast cancer

B Cervical cancer

C Endometrial cancer

D Ovarian cancer

For each of the descriptions, select the single most likely cancer. Each of the options may be used once, more than once, or not at all.

1 The most common malignant tumour that affects women only. ☐

2 Associated with an early menarche, rapid establishment of regular menstruation, obesity and high alcohol intake. ☐

3 Linked with unopposed oestrogen use; progestogen oral contraception may be protective. ☐

4 More common in nulliparous and subfertile women, and sometimes has a familial tendency. ☐

5 Linked with early teenage sexual intercourse, increased parity and smoking. ☐

6 Is usually a squamous carcinoma linked to oral contraceptive use over more than ten years. ☐

THEME: MENSTRUAL DISTURBANCES

A   Breakthrough bleeding

B   Cervical erosion

C   Climacteric

D   Endometriosis

E   Fibroids

F   Menorrhagia

G   Normal menstrual cycle

H   Pelvic inflammatory disease

I   Polycystic ovarian syndrome

For each patient with menstrual symptoms below, select the single most likely diagnosis. Each option may be used once, more than once, or not at all.

7   A 24-year-old woman with no previous gynaecological history of note complains of increased clear, non-offensive vaginal discharge and occasional post-coital spotting since restarting the Pill after her last pregnancy. She is otherwise asymptomatic. ☐

8   A 46-year-old woman complains that over the last 18 months her periods have been increasingly irregular, with intervals ranging from one week to six weeks between bleeds. Four months ago she was found to have a mild iron deficiency anaemia and she tells you that on occasion she floods. ☐

9   A 37-year-old Nigerian lady complains of heavy periods, urinary frequency and a progressive abdominal distension. ☐

10 A 36-year-old complains of a long history of dysmenorrhoea, deep dyspareunia and menorrhagia. She has come requesting referral for infertility. ☐

11 Miss Smith, a 22-year-old student consults you about her irregular cycles, which she says have been irregular for several years. Review of her records shows she has been seen in the past for dietary advice and has had Dianette® for acne. She is not currently taking any medications. ☐

12 A 22-year-old nurse complains that, since stopping the Pill, her periods have been irregular, usually two to three days early each month. ☐

THEME: CONTRACEPTION

A Combined pill

B Depo-Provera®

C Diaphragm

D HRT

E Implanon®

F Intra-uterine device insertion

G Levonelle-2®

H Minipill

I Mirena intra-uterine system

J Norplant®

K Sterilisation

L Triphasic pill

For each of the situations described below, select the most appropriate choice from the list above. Each answer may be used once, more than once, or not at all.

13 A 41-year-old woman attends for a routine Pill check. She is on Microgynon®. Review of her notes shows she has in the past tried barrier methods and fallen pregnant. She hates the thought of the coil. She is obese. Her blood pressure is 160/100 mmHg but she tells you that 'she has just run up the hill'. ☐

14 Miss Jones is leaving next week to spend nine months travelling around the world in her gap year. She does not have a boyfriend but would like something just in case. She is concerned about the risk of DVT. ☐

15 Late on Friday afternoon a 27-year-old mother of two comes to see you in surgery asking for contraception. After appropriate counselling you give her a prescription for Microgynon 30® to start at her next period. The following Tuesday she telephones you to say that she had intercourse on Friday night and would like the 'morning-after pill'. ☐

16 An 18-year-old student wants to go on the Pill. Review of her previous medical history shows she has in the past had migraines associated with numbness in her arms, although these are now controlled with ergotamine she often forgets to take it. ☐

17 At the Well Woman Clinic you see a woman who has not had a period for five months. Blood tests have shown that she is perimenopausal. She is in a stable sexual relationship and wants contraception but does not like the idea of the Pill. ☐

18 You see a 42-year-old woman who has suffered menorrhagia with flooding increasingly over the last two years. She has had minimal benefit from tranexamic acid but doesn't want a hysterectomy. She is currently on a combined oral contraceptive pill. ☐

MULTIPLE BEST ANSWER QUESTIONS

1 Select TWO of these statements about postnatal depression

☐ **A** Occurs in up to 25% of women after giving birth

☐ **B** Is more common in women with a history of psychiatric illness

☐ **C** Is more common in women who have had obstetric complications

☐ **D** Results in suicide attempts by up to 10% of affected women

☐ **E** Breast-feeding mothers with postnatal depression cannot be treated by antidepressant drugs because they are secreted into the breast milk in large amounts

2 Which THREE of the following statements about breast-feeding are true?

☐ **A** Foremilk contains more fat than hindmilk

☐ **B** Human milk is low in protein compared with cows' milk

☐ **C** Cows' milk and human milk have similar fat contents

☐ **D** Vitamin K levels are low in breast milk

☐ **E** An exclusively breast-fed baby's iron stores become low one month after birth

3 Select TWO of these items. Chlamydia infections

☐ **A** are asymptomatic in 25% of cases

☐ **B** do not usually affect subsequent fertility

☐ **C** can be tested for with urine samples

☐ **D** are the commonest curable STD in the developed world

☐ **E** are found in about 10% of the population

4   Select TWO statements about carcinoma of the cervix

☐ **A**   The majority of women with this have HPV infection

☐ **B**   The vast majority of women with HPV do not develop this

☐ **C**   Death rate is increasing

5   Select FOUR of the following items. Contraception using the combined oral contraceptive pill

☐ **A**   suppresses benign breast disease

☐ **B**   suppresses ovarian cysts

☐ **C**   decreases pelvic inflammatory disease

☐ **D**   decreases the incidence of ovarian cancer

☐ **E**   decreases the risk of arterial disease

☐ **F**   decreases the risk of breast cancer

6   Select TWO statements concerning hormonal post-coital contraception

☐ **A**   Must be used within 48 hours of unprotected sex

☐ **B**   Involves two doses spaced 12 hours apart

☐ **C**   Invariably contains oestrogens and progestogens

☐ **D**   Should be repeated 72 hours later if vomiting occurs

☐ **E**   Should be followed up if there is a delay of the next expected menstrual cycle

7   Antenatal women should be advised about which THREE of the following?

☐ **A** Take folic acid supplements for the first trimester

☐ **B** Take vitamin supplements, in particular vitamin A, for the first trimester

☐ **C** Take iron supplements throughout the pregnancy if iron deficient

☐ **D** Avoid all cheeses

☐ **E** Avoid all pâtés

8   THREE recognised causes of menorrhagia are

☐ **A** Thyrotoxicosis

☐ **B** Fibroids

☐ **C** Intra-uterine contraceptive device (IUCD)

☐ **D** Pelvic inflammatory disease

☐ **E** Anorexia

9   Which THREE of the following factors predispose to pre-eclampsia?

☐ **A** Diabetes

☐ **B** Multiparous women

☐ **C** Twin pregnancies

☐ **D** Hydatidiform mole

☐ **E** Myxoedema

10 Regarding contraception counselling for patients under 16, select TWO statements

☐ **A** They should always be accompanied by an adult

☐ **B** A full sexual history is not always essential

☐ **C** The combined oral contraceptive pill is often the most appropriate form of contraception

☐ **D** IUCDs can be inserted in a nulliparous patient

☐ **E** Mirena® is an option

11 Select THREE items which are true in relation to puerperal psychosis

☐ **A** Is much more common in primiparous women

☐ **B** Usually begins in the first two weeks after delivery

☐ **C** Recurrence in subsequent pregnancies is the rule

☐ **D** Usually has an insidious onset

☐ **E** Normally has a good prognosis

☐ **F** The most common presentation is a depressive illness

12 Choose TWO statements regarding perimenopausal contraception

☐ **A** FSH levels are reliable in women using the combined oral contraception pill

☐ **B** FSH levels are reliable in woman using the progesterone-only pill

☐ **C** A copper-containing IUD inserted at age 40 needs changing every three years

☐ **D** Mirena® is a possible form of contraception

13 Select THREE statements. Puerperal psychosis

☐ **A** usually begins within two days after childbirth

☐ **B** is commonly accompanied by clouding of consciousness

☐ **C** has a favourable prognosis

☐ **D** characteristically includes auditory hallucinations

☐ **E** characteristically includes obsessional ruminations

14 Choose THREE statements about torsion of the testis

☐ **A** Is most common in teenagers

☐ **B** Usually presents with abdominal pain and vomiting after trauma

☐ **C** Does not always require urgent referral

☐ **D** A non-viable testis should always be removed

☐ **E** An average General Practitioner is never likely to come across the condition

15 Select TWO items regarding benign prostatic hypertrophy

☐ **A** It is increasing in prevalence

☐ **B** Nocturia is a good diagnostic feature of the condition

☐ **C** Beta-blockers are the drugs of choice in managing mild conditions

☐ **D** The number of transurethral prostatectomy operations is increasing in the UK

☐ **E** It is essential to do a prostate-specific antigen (PSA) test once the condition is diagnosed

16 Select TWO of these statements concerning prostatic cancer

☐ **A** Is seldom seen in men under the age of 50

☐ **B** Is usually a poorly differentiated cancer

☐ **C** Can be accurately diagnosed using prostate-specific antigen

☐ **D** Can be treated by radiotherapy in the early stages as effectively as by surgery

☐ **E** Responds objectively in almost all cases to hormone therapy

SINGLE BEST ANSWER QUESTIONS

1   Select ONE statement that is NOT true about screening for prostate cancer

☐ **A**   PSA has a poor specificity

☐ **B**   PSA is a readily available test

☐ **C**   Some cancers detected by screening would never present clinically

☐ **D**   PSA can predict whether a cancer is dormant or aggressive

☐ **E**   Prostate biopsies may cause harm

2   Which ONE of the following is NOT true about childhood urinary tract infection?

☐ **A**   Has a benign outcome in most children

☐ **B**   Is diagnosed once culture of fresh urine yields pure bacterial growth of greater than 105 CFU/ml

☐ **C**   Is associated with vesico-ureteric reflux in two out of three affected children

☐ **D**   Is caused by an unsuspected surgical disorder in 5% of children

☐ **E**   Should be treated by combination antimicrobial therapy

3   Which ONE of the following is true with regard to breast cancer?

☐ **A**   The second most common cancer in women

☐ **B**   Incidence equates to a 1 in 25 lifetime risk for each woman

☐ **C**   Survival is improved by 15–20% by tamoxifen with oestrogen-receptor-positive tumours

☐ **D**   Treatment with tamoxifen has no effect on the risk of a further cancer in the other breast

☐ **E**   Screening with short intervals between screening episodes would prevent more deaths

4   Taking oral contraceptive steroids makes a woman more susceptible to which ONE of the following?

- ☐ **A**   Benign breast disease
- ☐ **B**   Carcinoma of the ovary
- ☐ **C**   Venous thrombosis
- ☐ **D**   Carcinoma of the uterus
- ☐ **E**   Pancreatitis

5   Which ONE of the following is true of endometrial cancer?

- ☐ **A**   It is more common among women using progestogen-containing oral contraceptives
- ☐ **B**   It is usually poorly differentiated
- ☐ **C**   It is now most effectively treated by a combination of radiotherapy and hormone-based chemotherapy
- ☐ **D**   It is characterised by late blood-borne metastasis, usually to the lung
- ☐ **E**   It has usually spread to local lymph glands at diagnosis

6   ONE medical factor considered in the use of the oral contraceptive pill is

- ☐ **A**   Progesterone-only preparations increase the blood pressure
- ☐ **B**   A previous history of arterial or venous thrombosis is a contraindication for a progesterone-only pill
- ☐ **C**   Combined preparations should be avoided in patients with sickle cell disease
- ☐ **D**   Malignant melanomas may be oestrogen dependent
- ☐ **E**   The progesterone-only pill is preferred in patients with epilepsy

7   Which ONE of the following statements best describes bladder cancer?

☐   **A**   Bladder cancer is usually a squamous carcinoma

☐   **B**   At presentation, most tumours have invaded the muscle of the bladder wall

☐   **C**   Survival correlates well with TNM staging at presentation

☐   **D**   Superficial tumours, if effectively treated by endoscopic resection and diathermy, seldom become invasive

☐   **E**   Chemotherapy for metastatic disease is ineffective and seldom used

8   Which ONE statement is true for prostate cancer?

☐   **A**   It is the second commonest cancer in men

☐   **B**   It is the commonest cause of cancer death in men

☐   **C**   It already has secondary spread in 10% at diagnosis in the UK

☐   **D**   Terminal events do not usually involve pain

☐   **E**   Screening does not appear to increase survival

SUMMARY COMPLETION QUESTION

THEME: ORAL CONTRACEPTIVE USE

Read the extract from the paper below, describing a study of Pill usage after the 1995 Pill scare, then read the commentary below. For each gap in the commentary, choose the most appropriate option from the list.

Influence of the third generation pill controversy on prescriptions for oral contraceptives among first time users: population based study. De Jogn van den Berg *et al British Medical Journal* 2003;326:254

Participants, methods and results

We used pharmacy dispensing data from the InterAction database (a general prescription drugs database) in the northern Netherlands. In 2000, the database contained prescriptions from a population of approximately 37, 000 women aged 15–44, and 224 prescribers (general practitioners and outpatient specialists). We selected all prescriptions for oral contraceptives from 1 January 1994 to 31 December 2000. First-time users of oral contraceptives were defined as women who, according to the database, either were prescribed any oral contraceptive for the first time or who had not been prescribed an oral contraceptive for at least one year. Hence, 1994 was used as a washout period. We calculated for first-time users of oral contraceptives the proportion of women per year receiving a third generation oral contraceptive (1995 to 2000). To study a change in the proportion, we used SPSS version 10 to calculate chi-squared tests for linear trend after stratification by age (>20, 20–24, 25–29, 30–34, 35–39, and ≥40 years).

The prevalence of women aged 15–44 taking the pill was stable from 1995 to 2000 (around 54%) (table). In 1995, the proportion of first-time oral contraceptive users taking a third generation pill was 73% for the youngest age group (15–20 years) and 65% for the women aged 20–24. For all other age groups, except for 30–34, the proportions were also above 50%, indicating that more than half of the first-time users received a third generation oral contraceptive. In 1996, the first year after the pill scare, the proportions decreased to below 50% for all age groups. The change was most evident in women younger than 20; for these users the percentage of all first-time users prescribed a third generation oral contraceptive decreased from 73% in 1995 to 11% in 2000.

Proportion of women taking a third generation oral contraceptive among first time users of oral contraceptives. Results are numbers (percentage)

	1995	1996	1997	1998	1999	2000	
Women aged 15-44 taking oral contraceptives	14, 862/27, 522 (54.0)	15, 914/29, 579 (53.8)	20, 529/37, 393 (54.9)	20, 417/37, 810 (54.0)	20, 201/37, 548 (53.8)	20, 086/37, 615 (53.4)	
Age of first time users (years):							
15-20	166/227 (73)	202/568 (36)	202/604 (33)	202/702 (29)	154/733 (21)	80/760 (11)	>0.001
20-24	129/200 (65)	104/237 (44)	79/202 (39)	94/262 (36)	60/225 (27)	49/220 (22)	>0.001
25-29	141/258 (55)	113/279 (41)	75/189 (40)	83/255 (33)	51/199 (26)	39/147 (27)	>0.001
30-34	102/222 (46)	85/261 (33)	68/217 (31)	78/229 (34)	55/196 (28)	54/163 (33)	0.006
35-39	71/138 (51)	61/182 (34)	37/150 (25)	50/210 (24)	55/193 (28)	28/153 (18)	>0.001
40-44	58/95 (61)	58/158 (37)	52/172 (30)	36/184 (20)	33/168 (20)	26/163 (16)	>0.001
Total	1140 (59)	1685 (37)	1534 (33)	1842 (30)	1714 (24)	1606 (17)	>0.001

Commentary

Third generation pills were a popular choice of contraception in the early 1990s, partly due to perceived beneficial cardiovascular effects. They were particularly popular for young and first-time users, and for many doctors soon became the drug of choice for hormonal contraception. Data linking the use of these drugs with increased____**(1)**____of thromboembolic disease resulted in many patients and their doctors turning away from these drugs. Anecdotal evidence over the following months suggested many users stopped the Pill altogether and the termination rate, the____**(2)**____outcome for failure of contraception, rose. This study looks at the after effects of this scare and aims to answer two questions: what happened to prescriptions for third generation pills and what happened to prescriptions for all pills?

The best way to monitor pill usage is to monitor pill____**(3)**____rather than____**(4)**____, avoiding____**(5)**____bias. The authors collected data for all prescriptions for a population of 37, 000 women from 224 prescribers. The scale of the population database should dilute any untoward influences from individuals, eg family planning clinics. They then analysed pill use according to age group and whether the pill user was a first-time user. This allows us to look at whether prescribing behaviour has changed for different groups of pill users.

The data reveal interesting results. Firstly the proportion of women receiving the pill stayed approximately the same between 1995 and 1996. The proportion receiving third generation pills fell significantly among all age groups between 1995 and 1996, and total pill prescribing has____**(6)**____. This is explained by the apparent increase in database size from 1995 through to 1997. Despite the increase in the____**(7)**____the____**(8)**____has outstripped this, reflected in the percentage of users on first-time scripts. The total proportion of women choosing the combined oral contraceptive is constant, suggesting the scare was limited to third generation pills, at least in the eyes of prescribers.

The authors do not explore the total number of third generation pill scripts issued. Was the change in prescribing behaviour limited to first-time users or all users. Those users with other risk factors (over 35 years old, smokers, overweight) are more at risk from thromboembolic effects and they should have seen large falls in prescriptions. The second area that would be interesting to follow up would be termination and birth rate over the corresponding period.

Options

A Prescribing

B Denominator

C Prevalence

D Population

E Incidence

F Levelled out

G Indicative

H Reporting

I Relative

J Surrogate

K Increased

L Declined

M Decreased

N Dispensing

O Numerator

P Compliance

RESPIRATORY MEDICINE

EXTENDED MATCHING QUESTIONS

THEME: BREATHLESSNESS

A Allergic alveolitis

B Asthma

C Hay fever

D Lung cancer

E Myocardial infarction

F Pulmonary embolism

For each patient with breathlessness, select the single most likely diagnosis. Each option can be used once, more than once, or not at all.

1 A 35-year-old non-smoking man presents with a 1-month history of breathlessness on exertion, especially in the mornings, productive cough, fever and weight loss of 3kg. He also complains of pains in his left leg following a fall in his aviary. Occasional crepitations were noted in the chest and his peak flow rate was 650 l/min. The left leg was not swollen but slightly tender over the calf. A chest X-ray showed fine nodularity. ☐

2 A 49-year-old female smoker presents with a short history of cough, haemoptysis and weight loss of 2kg. Peak flow was decreased but clinically the chest was clear. Chest X-ray showed opacity near the hilum. ☐

3 A 34-year-old male smoker presents with sore eyes, coryza, sneezing and breathlessness. His chest sounded wheezy and his recorded peak flow was 50% of that predicted for his age and height. Chest X-ray showed hyper-inflated lungs. ☐

4 A 34-year-old female smoker on the combined oral contraceptive pill presents with sudden onset of breathlessness and pain on the left side of the chest. On examination she is sweating profusely and is in pain and tachypnoeic. BP was normal. ☐

5 A 59-year-old male smoker presents with sudden-onset breathlessness and chest pains. On examination he is in pain, sweaty, has a tachycardia and BP is 90/50 mmHg.

THEME: BREATHLESSNESS

A Anaemia

B Asthma

C Bronchiectasis

D Chronic obstructive pulmonary disease (COPD)

E Inhalation of foreign body

F Laryngeal oedema

G Left ventricular failure

H Pleural effusion

I Pneumothorax

J Psychogenic breathlessness

K Pulmonary fibrosis

For each scenario described below, select the most likely diagnosis from the list above. Each option may be used once, more than once, or not at all.

6 A 77-year-old retired engineer complains of increasing breathlessness over several months. Examination reveals diffuse fine inspiratory crepitations and clubbing.

7 A 29-year-old woman being treated with clomiphene for infertility complains of increasing breathlessness and abdominal distension over the previous three weeks. She denies chest pain and has no previous respiratory history.

8 An 82-year-old lady with myelodysplasia has become progressively breathless over the last two weeks. Examination reveals tachycardia.

9 One summer's afternoon you are called to the beach where a trainee scuba diver has collapsed. She apparently complained of sudden left-sided pain on surfacing. When you arrive she is unconscious and tachypnoeic. Examination reveals reduced breath sounds on the left.

10 A three-year-old boy suddenly becomes breathless while eating at a children's party. When you examine him he is coughing and spluttering, with inspiratory wheeze. ☐

11 A 92-year-old lady is found extremely breathless in the middle of the night. She prefers to sit upright and on examination she has an irregular pulse, basal crepitations and is cyanosed. ☐

MULTIPLE BEST ANSWER QUESTIONS

1 Which TWO statements about childhood asthma are true?

☐ **A** Persistent cough may be the only symptom

☐ **B** About 50% of children will grow out of the disease

☐ **C** Outdoor exercises should be discouraged in winter months

☐ **D** Inhaled sodium chromoglycate is the drug of choice for prevention

☐ **E** Inhaled steroids normally stunt growth

2 When discussing smoking which TWO statements are true?

☐ **A** Non-smokers have a far greater risk of ischaemic heart disease if they live with a smoker

☐ **B** Nicotine replacement therapy is of no additional help in smoking cessation when the GP has given advice

☐ **C** The doctor–patient relationship may be harmed if the GP routinely advises all smokers to stop smoking

☐ **D** The increase in smoking is mostly because of the increasing elderly population

3 A severe asthma attack in an adult is characterised by which THREE indicators?

☐ **A** Restricted daily activities

☐ **B** Peak expiratory flow rate (PEFR) of 70% of predicted value

☐ **C** Pulse rate of 110 beats/minute

☐ **D** Difficulty in speaking

☐ **E** Peripheral cyanosis

4   Which TWO of the following are risk factors for the development of chronic obstructive pulmonary disease?

☐ **A**   Male sex

☐ **B**   Working with aniline dyes

☐ **C**   Low socioeconomic status

5   Which THREE statements apply to lung cancer?

☐ **A**   Causes deaths in the ratio 2:1, men to women, in the UK

☐ **B**   Is most prevalent among people aged over 70 years

☐ **C**   Is most commonly adenocarcinoma among smokers

☐ **D**   Has a clear genetic association

☐ **E**   Is associated with the level of urban pollution

6   What THREE common conditions cause increased resonance?

☐ **A**   Empyema

☐ **B**   Acute asthma

☐ **C**   Pneumothorax

☐ **D**   Emphysema

☐ **E**   Lung cancer

☐ **F**   Hyperventilation

SINGLE BEST ANSWER QUESTIONS

1 The British Thoracic Society guidelines for asthma indicate which ONE of the following?

☐ **A** Inhaled short acting beta-agonist should be given regularly as the first step

☐ **B** If inhaled short acting beta-agonists are needed more than once a day, an inhaled steroid should be used

☐ **C** Step three involves the addition of theophylline to beta-agonist tablet

☐ **D** Step four involves the addition of a long acting beta-agonist

2 Which ONE of the following is NOT a recognised association with finger clubbing?

☐ **A** Bronchiectasis

☐ **B** Emphysema

☐ **C** Lung cancer

☐ **D** Hepatic cirrhosis

☐ **E** Crohn's disease

3 Regarding the use of inhaled steroids in treatment, which ONE statement does NOT apply?

☐ **A** Side-effects are unusual at low doses

☐ **B** Indicated for children with episodic wheezing associated with viral illness

☐ **C** Systemic absorption takes place

☐ **D** Fluticasone may have fewer systemic side-effects than beclometasone

☐ **E** High dosage can slow growth in children

4   When considering treatment in chest infections, which ONE statement is true?

☐ **A**   25% of chest infections seen in General Practice are due to pneumonia

☐ **B**   50% of patients with lower respiratory tract infections receive antibiotics in General Practice

☐ **C**   Antibiotics should not be delayed in patients with COPD

5   Which ONE of the following statements about the investigations of asthma in children is true?

☐ **A**   Skin allergy tests are often diagnostic of the precipitating cause

☐ **B**   Chest radiographs are indicated whenever there is an acute episode

☐ **C**   Pulmonary function tests are useful in children over 2 years of age

☐ **D**   FEV1 is more reliable in demonstrating airways obstruction than peak expiratory flow

6   Which of these is NOT a recognised cause of cough?

☐ **A**   Inhaled foreign body

☐ **B**   Lisinopril

☐ **C**   Metformin

☐ **D**   Lung cancer

☐ **E**   Cardiac failure

7 Which ONE of these statements applies in the diagnosis of asthma?

☐ **A** 15% reversibility by bronchial dilators is an essential diagnostic test

☐ **B** Cough is an important diagnostic feature

☐ **C** Once diagnosed as asthmatics, children remain asthmatic for the rest of their lives

☐ **D** Steroid inhalers have an immediate bronchial dilator effect

☐ **E** Family history of asthma is irrelevant

8 Which ONE of the following statements does NOT apply to bronchial carcinoma?

☐ **A** Screening is of little benefit

☐ **B** It is more common in urban areas

☐ **C** Nickel is a recognised risk factor

☐ **D** The incidence in females is rising

☐ **E** Haemoptysis suggests a poor prognosis

9 In asthma which ONE of the following statements is true?

☐ **A** Mortality has been falling steadily over the past ten years

☐ **B** The long-acting inhaled bronchodilators are recommended for first-line therapy

☐ **C** Bacterial infections are a common cause of acute attacks

☐ **D** More than 90% of patients have hyper-reactive airways

☐ **E** Salbutamol and terbutaline act on adrenergic nerve endings to relax airway smooth muscle

PHOTO QUESTION

THEME: RESPIRATORY MEDICINE

For each image or results, select the desciption that is most likely to correspond to the history.

1 ☐

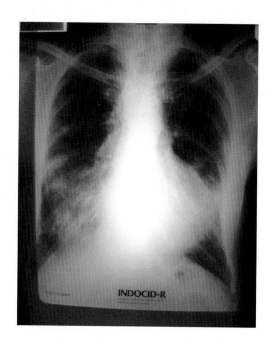

2 ☐

	Measured	Predicted	% Predicted
FVC	2.63	3.11	84
FEV1	1.28	2.28	56
FEV1/FVC	49	73	
FEF25-75	0.59	2.56	23
PEF	4.40	5.78	76

3 ☐

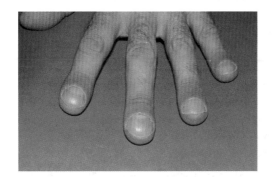

4 ☐

	Measured	Predicted	% Predicted
FVC	0.96	2.75	35
FEV1	0.94	1.90	49
FEV1/FVC	98	69	
FEF25-75	2.25	2.11	107
PEF	2.98	5.40	55

5 ☐

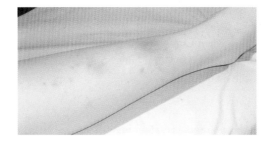

A A 3-month history of breathlessness, haemoptysis and weight loss.

B A 2-week history of cough and fever.

C Associated with hilar lymphadenopathy.

D A 7-year history of paroxysmal wheeze.

E A 60-year-old former coal miner with 18 months increasing dyspnoea and cough.

SUMMARY COMPLETION QUESTON

THEME: CHEST PAIN CLINIC

In an attempt to reduce the number of admissions with non-cardiac chest pain, your local District General Hospital decides to institute a chest pain clinic in A&E. The following paper describes an economic evaluation of such a scheme. Read the extract and the summary below, choosing appropriate options for each gap from the list.

Randomised controlled trial and economic evaluation of a chest pain observation unit compared with routine care. Goodacre *et al British Medical Journal* 2004;328:254–7

Abstract

Objectives To measure the effectiveness and cost effectiveness of providing care in a chest pain observation unit compared with routine care for patients with acute, undifferentiated chest pain.

Design Cluster randomised controlled trial, with 442 days randomised to the chest pain observation unit or routine care, and cost effectiveness analysis from a health service costing perspective.

Setting The emergency department at the Northern General Hospital, Sheffield, United Kingdom.

Participants 972 patients with acute, undifferentiated chest pain (479 attending on days when care was delivered in the chest pain observation unit, 493 on days of routine care) followed up until six months after initial attendance.

Methods

Intervention: chest pain observation unit

The chest pain observation unit was based in the emergency department and consisted of two monitored bays and an adjacent area for an unlimited number of unmonitored patients. It was staffed by three experienced (G grade) chest pain nurses with a background in either coronary care or emergency medicine, who had received additional training in supervising exercise treadmill tests. Together they

covered the chest pain observation unit from 9:00 am to 9:00 pm
Monday to Friday, and 10:00 am to 6:00 pm at weekends. Patients
attending outside these hours could be admitted and complete their
assessment the following day. Middle grade emergency department staff
provided medical cover. We selected patients according to validated
clinical predictors and offered assessment consisting of two to six hours
of ST segment monitoring and hourly electrocardiography, measurement
of biochemical cardiac markers (CKMB(mass) on arrival and at least two
hours later and of troponin T at least six hours after onset of symptoms)
and exercise treadmill testing. Patients with positive tests were admitted;
those with negative tests were discharged.

Control: routine care

Patients were managed at the discretion of the emergency department
medical staff, without use of the chest pain observation unit or
assistance from the chest pain nurses. The emergency department has
access to CKMB(mass) and troponin T assays with a turnaround time of
one hour. If patients required observation or further testing they were
admitted to hospital.

Reception staff (who were unaware of the randomisation schedule)
recorded the presenting complaint of all patients attending the
emergency department. The chest pain nurses then identified all
patients presenting with a specific list of chest pain related complaints
(prospectively when they were on duty and retrospectively, from a
computer generated list, at other times), and then excluded patients
with changes to their electrocardiogram that were diagnostic for acute
coronary syndrome, clinically diagnosed unstable angina, comorbidity,
or a serious alternative cause for chest pain; and patients who were
younger than 25, with a negligible risk of coronary heart disease, or
who were unable to take part in the trial or provide consent. Eligible
patients were asked to provide written, informed consent to subsequent
follow up. Those who declined to consent were still managed according
to availability of the chest pain observation unit but were not followed
up.

Follow up consisted of a clinic run by the chest pain nurses some 48
hours after initial attendance, at which an electrocardiogram was
recorded and troponin T concentration measured. Postal questionnaires
for completion by each patient were provided at 48 hours and one

month, for return to the medical care research unit. At six months we searched the hospital computer system for evidence of attendance at the emergency department or admission to hospital. We retrieved and reviewed relevant case notes. Finally, a research assistant telephoned each participant to collect further follow up information.

Main outcome measures The proportion of participants admitted to hospital, the proportion with acute coronary syndrome sent home inappropriately, major adverse cardiac events over six months, health utility, hospital reattendance and readmission, and costs per patient to the health service.

Results Use of a chest pain observation unit reduced the proportion of patients admitted from 54% to 37% (difference 17%, odds ratio 0.50, 95% confidence interval 0.39 to 0.65, $P<0.001$) and the proportion discharged with acute coronary syndrome from 14% to 6% (8%, −7% to 23%, $P = 0.264$). Rates of cardiac event were unchanged. Care in the chest pain observation unit was associated with improved health utility during follow up (0.0137 quality adjusted life years gained, 95% confidence interval 0.0030 to 0.0254, $P = 0.022$) and a saving of £78 per patient (−£56 to £210, $P = 0.252$).

Conclusions Care in a chest pain observation unit can improve outcomes and may reduce costs to the health service. It seems to be more effective and more cost effective than routine care.

Summary

Patients complaining of chest pain present both a clinical and economic____**(1)**____. How can we ensure that we ____**(2)**____ diagnostic sensitivity whilst we____**(3)**____ resource utilisation? This paper describes an economic evaluation of such a scheme implemented at a large metropolitan hospital. Patients presenting with chest pain were____**(4)**____into high, medium or low risk groups by the chest pain nurses. The medium risk group was then allocated to either routine care or chest pain observation unit. Randomisation was by day: the day of presentation was either a routine care day or a chest pain unit day, and all patients presenting on that day were treated accordingly. This process allows for adequate randomisation but due to the nature of triage and impossibility of blinding there is a strong possibility of selection bias by the chest pain nurse.

The primary outcome was the number of patients admitted to hospital, although it is not clear what the definition of admission is. One could argue that patients who present to the emergency department and are triaged to a chest pain observation unit where they stay for in excess of 6 hours for serial monitoring have effectively been admitted. This level of monitoring and presumably bed occupancy is likely to be comparable in cost to an admission. Secondary outcomes included cost, health utility and reattendance. In comparing the costs of the service it is not clear how the costs were calculated. Were the chest pain nurses____**(5)**____or was this a role taken on by the emergency department nurses, taking them away from their usual roles? Diversion of staff to a labour intensive observation unit will reduce their efficiency and ability to care for other patients, compared with usual care, where a patient with chest pain may be cared for by a nurse looking after other non-cardiac patients simultaneously. This reduced efficiency may have a deleterious effect on any apparent economic benefits.

The use of QALY and health utility indices may also be subject to bias. Since the study was un-blinded there may be____**(6)**____from the intensive observation and reassurance of the 'specialist nurse'. This may well modify____**(7)**____in future and enhance quality of life. Furthermore, the chest pain unit apparently had access to exercise treadmill testing, which was presumably not available to the routine care group without outpatient referral. Obviously this will reduce subsequent outpatient referrals for this investigation. It is unclear if this has been taken into consideration.

The results show a statistically____**(8)**____reduction in admissions, and ____**(9)**____cost saving in favour of the chest pain unit. These results ____**(10)**____support the implementation of such a system.

Options

A   Health seeking behaviour

B   Clearly

C   Minimise

D   Insignificant

E   Placebo effects

F   Dilemma

G   Attendances

H   Maximise

I   Puzzle

J   Attached

K   Diagnosed

L   Do not

M   Unequivocally

N   Triaged

O   Guardedly

P   Supernumerary

Q   Significant

R   Bias

SUMMARY COMPLETION QUESTION

THEME: COPD SCREENING

Your practice is seeking to reduce the impact of smoking-related diseases on your patient list. It has been suggested that you actively screen for chronic obstructive pulmonary disease (COPD) in these patients. While considering this issue you come across the following strategy which your practice nurse, who has recently completed a respiratory course, eagerly suggests you adopt.

Read the extract below and then the summary of the paper. For every blank response select the most appropriate response for the list below

Early detection of COPD in primary care: screening by invitation of smokers aged 40–55 years Stratelis et al British Journal of General Practice 2004;54:201–6.

Abstract

Aim To evaluate a method to detect COPD at an early stage in smokers in a young age group (40–55 years).

Design of study Prospective descriptive study.

Method

Population The study was performed in south-east Sweden, in the city of Motala (45, 000 inhabitants) and the surrounding suburban areas (43, 000 inhabitants). The population is served by nine primary healthcare centres. In the study area a total of 19, 750 inhabitants were between the age of 40 and 55 years. According to Swedish statistics, approximately 27% of this population in this age group are smokers.

Method Placards were displayed in each healthcare centre. An advertisement was placed in the local newspaper twice in the spring and twice in the autumn of one year (Box 1). The placards and advertisements invited smokers between the ages of 40 and 55 years to have a pulmonary function test (spirometry) performed free of charge, as well as giving the information that the aim of the test was to diagnose COPD at an early stage. Patients who already had a diagnosis of COPD were excluded from the study. Information about the relation between smoking and COPD was also given. A smoker was defined as someone who smoked at the time of the study or had stopped smoking less than 3 months before the study.

Pulmonary function testing The participants performed at least three dynamic spirometries during their visit to trained asthma and COPD nurses, all of whom had had at least 5 years' experience in the field. The spirometry was performed and interpreted according to the American Thoracic Society's recommendations. The results from all the spirometries performed by the nurses were re-evaluated by one experienced physician. If the spirometry was judged as not being optimal or showing obstruction, the participants were asked to perform another spirometry, performed by the same physician and using a Flowscreen version 3.10gb.

Results

A total of 512 smokers responded. The prevalence of COPD was 27% ($n = 141$). The COPD was classified as mild obstruction in 85% ($n = 120$), moderate in 13% ($n = 18$) and severe in 2% ($n = 3$) according to the European Respiratory Society classification. Knowledge of the disease COPD was acknowledged by 39% of the responders to the questionnaire. Logistic regression analysis showed that age, male sex, number of pack years, dyspnoea and symptoms of chronic bronchitis significantly increased the odds of having COPD. The adjusted odds ratio was significant for having >30 pack years.

Conclusions

This method of inviting relatively young smokers selected from a population of smokers with a high incidence of COPD, may be one way of identifying smokers with COPD in the early stages from the list following the summary.

Summary

The_____**(1)**_____ of this methodology to United Kingdom general practice is_____**(2)**_____ in assessing whether such a model could work here: to decide this we need to answer the following questions. Firstly, is the study population broadly similar_____**(3)**_____ to our own, and secondly is the healthcare system similar to our own. The first point relates principally to the demographics of the study population: are they of a similar age:sex and economic group and do they have a similar standard of living? COPD is related both to smoking and to occupational exposure to certain chemicals. Comparison of a group of upper middle class stockbrokers in leafy suburbs with the inhabitants of a former colliery town in south Wales will clearly show vastly different _____(4)_____ and also the health beliefs of the populations will be different. As important is the ethnic background of the population, which may affect both disease rates and response to interventions, particularly_____(5)_____ health promotion.

The healthcare system in the study population is also important in assessing the relevance of the study to our practice. In a society where healthcare is free at the point of contact, as in the NHS, the offer of free screening may be seen as of low priority, when patients can be seen and treated for free when the disease manifests itself clinically. On the other hand, in a country where the user pays for any intervention or contact, the offer of free screening which will potentially offer great improvements in long term health and hence healthcare costs is likely to be warmly received.

The intervention is undoubtedly successful in increasing the diagnosis of early and pre-COPD in previously undiagnosed patients. However, the costs need to be considered. The large sums of money which need to be spent to promote the service may well represent a significant _____(6)_____ to the system. The diversion of these resources may result in fewer resources being available for other interventions, eg medications such as_____(7)_____ or pulmonary rehabilitation schemes. There is abundant evidence that_____(8)_____ screening and health promotion is a more cost-effective intervention, since patients who are currently suffering from a smoking-related illness have a greater motivation to change. Targeting all smokers on a practice list would also be another effective strategy, since the intervention would be specifically aimed at the relevant group, rather than a blanket scheme aimed at 100% of the population despite the fact that only 27% of them smoke.

The final issue that this study does not address is long-term _____(9)_____. Does screening and diagnosis of COPD in this group of patients result in improvement in morbidity and mortality. The only intervention which effects long-term survival is _____(10)_____. This study does not tell us if

157

the system in place results in any significant reduction in smoking rates in this group.

Options

A   Socioeconomically

B   Smoking cessation

C   Pro-active

D   Applicability

E   Tiotropium

F   Outcome

G   Vital

H   Targeted

I   Morbidity

J   Random

K   Opportunity cost

L   Beta-2 agonists

M   Steroids

N   Reactive

O   Pathology

ADMINISTRATION AND MANAGEMENT QUESTIONS

ADMINISTRATION AND MANAGEMENT

EXTENDED MATCHING QUESTIONS

THEME: CONSULTATION: WRITERS, MODELS AND THEORIES

A   Biomedical model

B   Balint

C   Berne

D   Byrne and Long

E   Heron

F   Neighbour

G   Pendleton, Schofield, Tate and Havelock

H   Rosenstock, Becker and Maiman

I   Stott and Davis

Choose one of the above options for each of the following statements. Each option may be used once, more than once, or not at all.

1 Identifies three ego states. ☐

2 Mentions six category intervention model. ☐

3 Involves the classical medical diagnostic process. ☐

4 Mentions management of presenting and continuing problems, as well as changing help-seeking behaviour and opportunistic health promotion. ☐

5 Relies on an objective medical disorder being found, and does not consider the doctor–patient relationship. ☐

6 Involves consultation mapping. ☐

7 Uses the terms doctor-centred and patient-centred, and analysed thousands of tape-recorded consultations. ☐

THEME: LEGISLATION

A   Access to Health Records Act 1990

B   Access to Medical Reports Act 1988

C   Data Protection Act 1984

D   Disability Discrimination Act 1995

E   Rehabilitation of Offenders Act 1974

For each of the descriptions, select the single most likely Act. Each option may be used once, more than once, or not at all.

 8 After a certain length of time, criminal convictions must not be mentioned in any reports.

 9 Patients can see any reports prepared for insurance companies.

10 Allows patients to see their own medical notes.

11 Gives employers responsibilities in relation to employees who have previously been disabled.

12 Ensures that personal data are only held for specific purposes.

THEME: VOLUNTARY ORGANISATIONS

A   Alanon

B   ASH

C   Compassionate Friends

D   CRUSE

E   Gingerbread

F   Marie Curie Memorial Foundation

G   MIND

H   NSPCC

I   RELATE

J   RNIB

K   RSPB

L   RSPCA

M   Terrence Higgins Trust

N   Turning Point

For each of the situations, select the single most appropriate organisation. Each option may be used once, more than once, or not at all.

13 Blindness. ☐

14 Widows with bereavement problems. ☐

15 Marriage problems. ☐

16 Mental illness. ☐

17 AIDS. ☐

18 Bereaved parents. ☐

19 Relatives of people with alcohol problems. ☐

20 Child abuse. ☐

21 One-parent families. ☐

22 Cancer. ☐

23 Children suffering bereavement problems after death of parents. ☐

24 Smokers. ☐

25 Drug abuse. ☐

THEME: NUMBERS OF PEOPLE ON A GP'S LIST

A 5

B 10

C 25

D 50

E 100

F 200

For each of the groups of people below, select the single most likely numbers. Each option may be used once, more than once, or not at all.

26 Number of unemployed people. ☐

27 Number of schizophrenic patients. ☐

28 Number of deaf people. ☐

29 Number of people receiving state benefits. ☐

30 Number of blind people. ☐

THEME: MEDICAL CERTIFICATES

A   Med 3

B   Med 4

C   Med 5

D   Med 6

E   Med 10

F   DS 1500

For each of the descriptions, select the single most likely medical certificate. Each option may be used once, more than once, or not at all.

31 Issued when a vague diagnosis has been given on a certificate. ☐

32 Is the usual certificate issued by a medical practitioner if a patient is off work because of sickness for more than seven days. ☐

33 Is issued by a hospital if a patient is to be off work due to illness. ☐

34 Is issued about a patient who has a terminal illness. ☐

35 Is issued at the patient's request when personal capability assessment is being considered. ☐

36 Can be issued for up to six months when the patient is first off work with an illness. ☐

37 Can be issued as a sickness certificate on the basis of a written report from another doctor. ☐

MULTIPLE BEST ANSWER QUESTIONS

1   Select TWO of the following about a learning portfolio

☐ **A**   Includes your hobbies

☐ **B**   Is a useful tool when looking for jobs outside medicine

☐ **C**   Is a record of past experience and future plans

☐ **D**   Could include audit, research projects and patient surveys

☐ **E**   Needs to be kept in hard copy

☐ **F**   Needs to be typed

2   Select TWO correct statements about GPs complaints procedure

☐ **A**   All GPs must operate a practice-based complaints procedure

☐ **B**   GPs can opt to use a PCT-based complaint procedure

☐ **C**   The procedure must be practice owned

☐ **D**   The procedure must be supported by a clear majority of staff

☐ **E**   The procedure can be sufficiently publicised with oral
           information from the staff

3   Select TWO of the following statements. A competent adult:

☐ **A**   Cannot refuse treatment if the treatment is indicated

☐ **B**   Cannot refuse treatment if death would result

☐ **C**   Cannot refuse treatment if it would be detrimental to a fetus

☐ **D**   Retains information long enough to allow an effective decision

☐ **E**   Understands the nature and purpose of treatment, including
           the risks, benefits and the alternatives

4   Select TWO of the following items about consulting by email

☐   **A**   Likely to lessen workload

☐   **B**   Avoids problems with GMC and medical defence organisations

☐   **C**   Can be used to help book appointments

☐   **D**   Patients might make contact from abroad

☐   **E**   Encouraged by the GMC and GP committees

5   The new contract of 2003 involves which TWO of the following?

☐   **A**   The contract is between the GP and Primary Care Trust (PCT)

☐   **B**   All practices must cover the provision of health care to everyone who believes themselves to be ill

☐   **C**   The care of violent patients is a directed enhanced service

☐   **D**   Cryosurgery is considered to be minor surgery

☐   **E**   All practices are required to offer contraceptive care

6   Select TWO of the following statements about revalidation

☐   **A**   The GMC expects about 60% of doctors to be recommended for revalidation

☐   **B**   Applies only to NHS doctors

☐   **C**   Involves good clinical care

☐   **D**   Requires doctors to sign declarations about their own health and probity

☐   **E**   Is a 10-yearly exercise

7   Which TWO of the following are NOT arguments in favour of the independent contractor status of GPs?

☐ **A** Allows a flexible way of working

☐ **B** Means that doctors do not need to worry about money

☐ **C** Means doctors do not need to be ruled by PCTs and can ignore NSFs

☐ **D** Allows greater control of their jobs, eg staff

☐ **E** Means they can act independently on behalf of patients

8   Which TWO of the following CANNOT give consent for a child

☐ **A** Child's mother if not married at the time of conception or birth

☐ **B** Child's father if not married at the time of conception or birth

☐ **C** Child's younger brother or sister

☐ **D** Person holding a residence order from a court

☐ **E** A local authority designated in a court order

9   Select THREE restrictions with respect to driving which apply to patients at risk of having seizures

☐ **A** Patients are obliged to contact the DVLA if they believe themselves to be at risk of seizures

☐ **B** A patient's doctor is obliged to inform the DVLA of a patient at risk of seizures

☐ **C** A patient may continue to drive following a single nocturnal seizure

☐ **D** A recent diagnosis of cerebral glioma prohibits driving

☐ **E** A recent diagnosis of bronchogenic carcinoma prohibits driving

10 **Select TWO occupations suitable for someone with a history of epilepsy, but who has not had a fit for the last five years**

☐ **A** An aircraft pilot

☐ **B** A prison officer

☐ **C** A teacher

☐ **D** A train driver

☐ **E** An army officer

☐ **F** A merchant seafarer

11 **Select THREE of the following. Burnout in General Practitioners is**

☐ **A** More likely to be found in doctors with postgraduate qualifications

☐ **B** Less likely in those who attend postgraduate meetings

☐ **C** Unrelated to depression

☐ **D** More likely in doctors with obsessional personalities

☐ **E** More likely in those with high personal standards

☐ **F** Less likely in those who are reluctant to delegate at work

12 **Select THREE factors concerning heartsink patients**

☐ **A** Doctors with postgraduate medical qualifications have more heartsink patients

☐ **B** Doctors trained in counselling have more heartsink patients

☐ **C** The more heartsink patients seen, the lower the job satisfaction

☐ **D** Heartsink patients have high rates of non-attendance for appointments

☐ **E** About one-third of heartsink patients have a serious medical diagnosis

13 **Which THREE of the following are available as over-the-counter medicines and do not need a doctor's prescription?**

☐ **A** Cimetidine

☐ **B** Piroxicam tablets

☐ **C** Ibuprofen tablets

☐ **D** Topical aciclovir

☐ **E** Co-proxamol

14 **Free NHS prescriptions are available to which THREE groups of patients?**

☐ **A** All patients with thyrotoxicosis

☐ **B** All patients with myasthenia gravis

☐ **C** All patients with diabetes

☐ **D** Patients with a permanent fistula

☐ **E** Patients with epilepsy

15 **Select THREE statements about advance directives**

☐ **A** Once made, cannot be withdrawn

☐ **B** Need to state that death might result from the directive

☐ **C** Must not be deliberately ignored

☐ **D** Need to be signed and witnessed

☐ **E** Can stop the administration of oral nutrition and hydration

16 On confirmation of death, one needs to inform the coroner about which THREE of these situations?

☐ **A** Patient was not seen in the previous 14 days

☐ **B** Death followed a termination of pregnancy

☐ **C** Patient has had chemotherapy in the last month

☐ **D** Patient has a pacemaker fitted

☐ **E** Death was due to an industrial disease

17 Select the THREE items which can be prescribed on FP10

☐ **A** Viagra® tablets

☐ **B** Pen insulin injection devices

☐ **C** Neck collar

☐ **D** Blood pricking lancets

☐ **E** Panadol®

18 A patient requests access to their records. Which TWO of the following are true?

☐ **A** Paper notes about an individual are the legal property of that individual

☐ **B** Under the Medical Records Act 1988 a doctor must amend a report before sending it if the patient disagrees with it

☐ **C** If a patient requests a copy of a medical report, the practice may make a charge for this

☐ **D** Medical records must be divulged in full should a patient request this

☐ **E** Patients may view a copy of the report up to six months after it has been written

☐ **F** Medical records are exempt from the Data Protection Act

☐ **G** GPs may only charge for access to paper records, not computer records

SINGLE BEST ANSWER QUESTIONS

1   PMS was set up to for which ONE of the following reasons

☐ **A**   Give personal service and avoid a nurse led service

☐ **B**   Unify contracts with the PCT

☐ **C**   Increase the independent role of a GP

☐ **D**   Guarantee budgets

☐ **E**   Attract GPs to areas of recruitment problems

2   Select ONE item about a practice that becomes a training practice

☐ **A**   The workload for the partners is likely to reduce

☐ **B**   The patients should be informed

☐ **C**   The partners' views on organisational matters will be accepted

☐ **D**   The deanery will organise any special equipment, eg video, that is needed

☐ **E**   The registrar can be excluded from all practice meetings

3   Select ONE of the following about the new contract of 2003

☐ **A**   All money is for quality

☐ **B**   The Carr Hill formula applies to quality

☐ **C**   Quality payments are not made via the PCT

☐ **D**   There are two quality domains: one for clinical aspects and one for organisational aspects

☐ **E**   Quality payment includes essential and enhanced services

4   Choose ONE of the following. Self-regulation

☐ **A**   Is about a doctor deciding what he/she is going to do

☐ **B**   Is about the profession deciding on its own codes of ethics and behaviour

☐ **C**   Is not possible with a better-informed public

☐ **D**   Allows the profession to protect its own interests

☐ **E**   Is enhanced by loss of public confidence

5   Which ONE of these is NOT true about the new contract for GPs?

☐ **A**   Less chance to get a salaried position

☐ **B**   Possible to opt out of 24-hour responsibility

☐ **C**   Seniority payments start earlier

☐ **D**   PCT will purchase all it equipment

☐ **E**   Pensions will improve

6   Select ONE of the following. Personal Development Plans

☐ **A**   Are a plan from the PCT

☐ **B**   Will be financially rewarded

☐ **C**   Involve regular exercise and healthy eating

☐ **D**   Are given to all suitable patients

☐ **E**   Require learning portfolios for all members of the practice team

7   Most commercial flights will allow pregnant women to fly on
     board up to which ONE of the gestational periods given below?

☐   **A**   38 weeks

☐   **B**   34 weeks

☐   **C**   30 weeks

☐   **D**   26 weeks

8   A 32-year-old lady with an established diagnosis of bipolar
     affective disorder is visited regularly by an outreach team. The
     team is increasingly concerned about her self-care since she
     stopped taking her mood-stabilising drugs. If she needs to be
     detained in hospital, which SINGLE section of the Mental Health
     Act (1983) would be the MOST appropriate?

☐   **A**   Section 2

☐   **B**   Section 3

☐   **C**   Section 4

☐   **D**   Section 5

☐   **E**   Section 7

9   Which ONE of the following would the General Medical Council
     NOT expect a doctor to do?

☐   **A**   Be actively supportive of the professional development of each
            member of their practice team

☐   **B**   Report another doctor immediately if patients are at risk of
            harm

☐   **C**   Meet performance targets set by management

☐   **D**   Disclose personal information about a patient if this is in the
            wider public interest, after weighing up the harm and benefit

☐   **E**   Be prepared to explain and justify their decisions

ADMINISTRATION AND MANAGEMENT

10 With regard to complaints made to a practice, which ONE of the following statements is true?

☐ **A**   The time limit for a patient to lodge a complaint is six months

☐ **B**   Complaints must be acknowledged within seven working days

☐ **C**   The senior partner is responsible for the administration of the complaints system

☐ **D**   90% of practice complaints are because of rudeness or other interpersonal issues

☐ **E**   There must be a written response within ten working days

RESEARCH, EPIDEMIOLOGY AND STATISTICS

RESEARCH, EPIDEMIOLOGY AND STATISTICS

EXTENDED MATCHING QUESTIONS

THEME: ORLISTAT

A 1

B 2

C 2.5

D 3

E 5

F 6

G 10

H 15

I 25

J 28

K 30

L 32

M 35

N Breathlessness

O Aerobics

P Dietary

Q Will power

R Activity

S Hypothyroidism

T Hypertension

U Gastro-oesophageal reflux

From the list of options, select the appropriate word for each gap.
Each option may be used once, more than once, or not at all.

The National Institute for Clinical Excellence has recommended that
orlistat should be prescribed under the following conditions:

- Only for individuals with a body mass index (BMI)
  of ____(1)____ kg/m² or more (and no associated co-morbidity)
  or for individuals with a BMI of ____(2)____ kg/m² or more in
  the presence of other risk factors (eg type 2 diabetes,
  ____(3)____, hypercholesterolaemia).

- Only for individuals who have lost at least ____(4)____ kg
  body weight by____(5)____control and increased____(6)____
  in the preceding month.

- Only for individuals aged between 18 and 75 years.

- Treatment should continue beyond three months only if
  weight loss is greater than ____(7)____ % from start of
  treatment.

- Treatment should continue beyond ____(8)____ months only if
  weight loss is greater than ____(9)____ % from start of
  treatment.

- Treatment should not usually continue beyond ____(10)____
  year(s) and never beyond____(11)____ year(s).

THEME: STATISTICS

A 112/183

B 112/175

C 112/1000

D 71/183

E 71/825

F 71/1000

G 63/175

H 63/817

I 63/1000

J 754/817

K 754/825

L 754/1000

One thousand patients were tested in General Practice for colonic cancer using a new test. The test was positive in 112 patients who actually had the disease, and in 71 patients who did not have the disease. The test was negative in 63 patients who actually did have the disease and in 754 patients who did not have the disease. For each of the statements, select the single most likely option. Each option can be used once, more than once, or not at all.

12 What is the sensitivity? ☐

13 What is the positive predictive value? ☐

14 What is the negative predictive value? ☐

15 What is the specificity? ☐

THEME: TRIALS

A   Case–control study

B   Cohort study

C   Correlation study

D   Descriptive study

E   Meta-analysis study

F   Randomised clinical trial

G   Randomised crossover trial

H   Randomised double-blind placebo-controlled trial

For each description below, select the single most likely study. Each option may be used once, more than once, or not at all.

16   A survey to find the prevalence of diabetes in a General Practice population. ☐

17   A study looking at the previous use of aspirin in patients with deep vein thromboses (DVTs) and in healthy patients. ☐

18   The prevention of DVTs was studied in air travellers who were assigned randomly to receive either stockings or exercise. ☐

19   Reported national incidence of psychotic illness is found to be associated with the national seizure of illicit drugs. ☐

20   The results of several investigations into exposure to vibrating machinery and the development of hand-arm vibration syndrome are combined to reach a conclusion. ☐

THEME: STATISTICAL TERMS

A   0

B   1

C   Just over 1

D   Just under 2

E   2

F   Just over 2

G   Just under 3

H   3

I   Over 3

The number of receptionists employed by General Practices in a local area were as follows: 1, 2, 0, 7, 0, 4, 2, 2, 1, 1, 2. For each of the questions, select the single most likely option. Each option can be used once, more than once, or not at all.

21   What is the mean?   ☐

22   What is the median?   ☐

23   What is the mode?   ☐

THEME: ECONOMICS

A Cost

B Cost-benefit analysis

C Cost-benefit ratio

D Cost-effective

E Cost-effectiveness analysis

F Cost-effectiveness ratio

G Cost-minimisation analysis

H Cost-of-illness analysis

I Cost-utility analysis

J Price

For each of the statements, select the single most likely option. Each of the options can be used once, more than once, or not at all.

24 A type of economic assessment in which both cost and benefit are expressed in monetary terms.

25 The monetary value of the resources consumed in production or delivery.

26 The ratio of total cost of an intervention divided by the gain in selected health outcome (eg cost per life/year gained).

27 A study to estimate the economic burden of a particular disease.

28 A study to assess the benefit of an intervention, eg quality-adjusted life-year.

THEME: STUDIES

A   Case–control study

B   Cohort study

C   Correlation study

D   Descriptive study

E   Meta-analysis study

F   Randomised double-blind crossover trial

G   Randomised double-blind placebo-controlled trial

For each of the scenarios listed below select the most appropriate type of study. Each option may be use once, more than once, or not at all.

29 A group of children using mobile phones was matched with a group only using land-based phones. The groups were both followed up, looking at the incidence of brain tumours. ☐

30 Patients with osteoarthritis were randomly given drug A or drug B, which looked identical. The clinical condition was monitored. The patients were then given the alternative drug and monitored again. Neither the doctor nor the patient knew which drug was being taken at each time. ☐

31 Patients with warts were randomly given preparation X in a paste base, or the paste base alone. The warty lesions were observed. Neither the doctor nor the patient knew which treatment was being given. ☐

32 A group of patients with DVTs was matched with a healthy group of people of the same age, sex and social class. It was then established how often they had travelled by plane in the past year. ☐

33 A group of diabetics was investigated to see if the mothers had had certain infections during their pregnancies. ☐

THEME: SCREENING TESTS

A   0.2

B   0.8

C   20%

D   25%

E   33%

F   50%

G   66%

H   80%

I   93%

In a sample of 100 undergoing a screening test, there were 20 true positives, 5 false negatives, 5 false positives and 70 true negatives. For each option, select the single most likely figure. Each option may be used once, more than once, or not at all.

34 Sensitivity.   ☐

35 Specificity.   ☐

36 Prevalence.   ☐

37 Predictive value.   ☐

38 Yield.   ☐

THEME: RESEARCH METHODS

A   Clinical audit

B   Longitudinal study

C   Observational study

D   Qualitative study

E   Randomised controlled trial

F   Survey

For each of the statements, select the single most likely option. Each option can be used once, more than once, or not at all.

39 A General Practice wishes to see how it manages its diabetic patients as compared to other practices in the area. ☐

40 A Health Authority wishes to know how many of its black African population are screened for sickle-cell disease. ☐

41 A General Practice wishes to explore the views of women who do not wish to breast-feed. ☐

42 A GP wishes to find out if salbutamol inhaler is less effective than brand-named Ventolin®. ☐

43 An occupational health doctor wishes to find out if telling the factory workers they have hypertension leads to more time off sick. ☐

THEME: STATISTICAL TERMS

A   Sensitivity

B   Sensitivity analysis

C   Significance levels

D   Specificity

E   Standard deviation

F   Standard error of the mean (SEM)

G   Standard normal variant

H   Standardised mortality rate

For each of the statements, select the single most likely option. Each option can be used once, more than once, or not at all.

44 A term used for describing recomputation of results using different parameters, values or perspectives to investigate whether any conclusions drawn are altered as a result. ☐

45 A measure of the spread of a distribution and is equal to the square root of the variance. ☐

46 The true-positive ratio, that is the proportion of patients with disease who return a positive test. ☐

47 Widely used statistic to describe the precision associated with the estimate of the mean. ☐

48 Mortality rate adjusted to take account of the composition of the population to which it refers. ☐

THEME: LITERATURE IN GENERAL PRACTICE

A   Balint M. *The Doctor, his Patient and the Illness*. London: Tavistock, 1958

B   Berne E. *Transactional Analysis – Games People Play*. London: Penguin, 1970

C   Byrne PS, Long BEL. *Doctors Talking to Patients*. London: DHSS, 1976

D   Heron J. *Human Potential Research Project*. University of Surrey, 1975

E   Neighbour R. *The Inner Consultation*. Petroc Press, 1999

F   Pendleton D. *The Consultation*. Oxford: Oxford University Press, 1984

G   Stott CP, Davis RH. The exceptional potential in each primary care consultation. *Journal of the Royal College of General Practitioners* 1979; **29**: 201–15

Each of the following comments relate to consultation texts above. Select the single most likely reference. Each option can be used once, more than once, or not at all.

49 The seven tasks. ☐

50 Modification of help-seeking behaviour. ☐

51 Six logical phases to a consultation. ☐

52 Doctor as drug. ☐

53 The achievement of a shared understanding of the problems with the patient. ☐

54 Parent, adult and child ego states. ☐

55 Cathartic. ☐

56 Opportunistic health promotion. ☐

57 Safety-netting. ☐

58 Apostolic function. ☐

THEME: A YEAR IN GENERAL PRACTICE

A   500

B   200

C   25

D   10

E   <1

For each of the conditions, select the most likely number of patients consulting with each condition. Each option may be used once, more than once, or not at all.

59 Chronic renal failure. ☐

60 Chronic mental illness. ☐

61 Hypertension. ☐

62 Thyroid disease. ☐

63 Diabetes. ☐

THEME: TRIALS CONCERNING CORONARY HEART DISEASE

A 4S

B ASSET

C CARE Study

D GISSI

E GREAT Group Study

F ISIS-2

G Nurses Study

For each description below, select the most likely trial. Each option may be used once, more than once, or not at all.

64 A trial of thrombolytic therapy using streptokinase controlled against placebo. ☐

65 A trial of pre-hospital thrombolytic treatment. ☐

66 This trial used simvastatin. ☐

67 This was a large-scale trial of lipid-lowering drugs in secondary prevention; pravastatin was the active drug used. ☐

68 A trial of thrombolytic therapy using aspirin and/or streptokinase. ☐

69 This study involved the use of unopposed oestrogens. ☐

70 Trial of a thrombolytic which used therapy. ☐

THEME: CARDIOVASCULAR TRIALS

A 4S

B Antiplatelet Trialists' Collaboration 94

C CARE

D HOPE

E HOT

F ISIS-2

G SOLVD-T

H UKPDS-1998

I WOSCOPS

For each of the following descriptions of clinical trials, choose the corresponding trial from the list above. Each option may be used once, more than once, or not at all.

71 Confirmed the value of primary prevention in preventing cardiovascular deaths in patients with hyperlipidaemia. ☐

72 Confirmed the value of treating post-MI patients with left ventricular dysfunction with ACE inhibitors. ☐

73 Showed the benefit of secondary prevention in patients with ischaemic heart disease with normal lipid levels. ☐

74 Confirmed the value of immediate aspirin after MI. ☐

75 Confirmed that the ideal BP in terms of reducing cardiovascular complications is 140/80 mmHg. ☐

76 Confirmed the value of tight control of blood pressure in diabetes mellitus. ☐

THEME: HYPERTENSION

A 5

B 10

C 15

D 85

E 90

F 100

G 100

H 110

I 145

J 150

K 160

L ACE inhibitors

M Aspirin

N Beta-blockers

O Clopidogrel

P Fibrates

Q Non-pharmacological measures

R Pharmacological measures

S Statins

T Thiazides

Below is a summary of the British Hypertension Society Guidelines (2000). For each omitted item, select the most appropriate option from the list above.

Use_____**(77)**_____in all hypertensive and borderline hypertensive people. Initiate antihypertensive drug treatment in people with sustained systolic blood pressure 160 mmHg or sustained diastolic blood pressure of _____**(78)**_____mmHg. Decide on treatment in people with sustained systolic blood pressure between 140 and 159 mmHg or sustained diastolic blood pressure between 90 and 99 mmHg according to the presence or absence of target organ damage, cardiovascular disease, diabetes, or a 10-year coronary heart disease risk of_____**(79)**_____%

according to the Joint British Societies coronary heart disease risk
assessment programme or risk chart. Optimal blood pressure treatment
targets are systolic blood pressure <____**(80)**____mmHg and diastolic
blood pressure <____**(81)**____mmHg; the minimum acceptable level of
control (audit standard) recommended is <____**(82)**____/<____**(83)**____
mmHg. In the absence of contraindications or compelling indications
for other antihypertensive agents,____**(84)**____or____**(85)**____are
preferred as first-line treatment for the majority of hypertensive people;
compelling indications and contraindications for all antihypertensive
drug classes are specified. Other drugs that reduce cardiovascular risk
must also be considered: these include____**(86)**____and____**(87)**____.

MULTIPLE BEST ANSWER QUESTIONS

1 **Select THREE of these statements concerning the mental health of children and adolescents in Great Britain**

☐ **A** 10% of 5- to 15-year-olds have a clinically significant mental disorder

☐ **B** More girls are affected than boys

☐ **C** More children are affected in families with both parents working

☐ **D** 30% of children with a mental disorder have no contact with General Practice or specialist services

☐ **E** These children are three times more likely to have special educational needs

2 **Select TWO statements that relate most to children in social class V compared with social class I**

☐ **A** Are four times more likely to die in an accident

☐ **B** Are taller in height

☐ **C** Have the same rate of chronic illness

☐ **D** Have a much higher infant mortality rate

3 **Select TWO of the following statements regarding obesity in the UK**

☐ **A** Is increasing in prevalence

☐ **B** Is more common in social class I compared to social class V

☐ **C** Should be treated with pharmacological intervention when the BMI is 29 kg/m^2

☐ **D** The body fat distribution in the South Asian population is the same as that in the white population

☐ **E** Is an independent risk factor for hypertension

4 **The risk of dying from liver cirrhosis is higher than average in which TWO groups?**

- [ ] **A** Farm workers
- [ ] **B** Journalists
- [ ] **C** Medical practitioners
- [ ] **D** Printing machine minders
- [ ] **E** Managers in the building and contracting trade

5 **When comparing retrospective studies to prospective studies, select THREE statements relating to retrospective studies**

- [ ] **A** More prone to bias
- [ ] **B** More expensive
- [ ] **C** Less attributable to cause and effect
- [ ] **D** Quicker to do
- [ ] **E** More rigorous

6 **In the trial of two anti-epileptic drugs following head injury, 18 out of 27 patients treated by drug A were fit-free one month after injury compared with 5 out of 17 patients treated with drug B. Select THREE of the following statements which apply if the significance of these results is tested by the chi-squared test**

- [ ] **A** The figures should first be converted to percentages
- [ ] **B** The test is non-parametric
- [ ] **C** There is one degree of freedom
- [ ] **D** A chi-squared value of 4.3 would imply that the result would have been obtained by chance in 43 out of 100 trials
- [ ] **E** The results would be invalidated if most of the cases treated with drug A had developed epilepsy immediately after the head injury compared with those treated with drug B

7 Select THREE of the following statements about systematic reviews

☐ **A** Are dependent on having good randomised controlled trials

☐ **B** Odds ratios and associated 95% confidence intervals are usually reported

☐ **C** Are available for most medical interventions

☐ **D** Are routinely used by commissioners to make purchasing decisions

☐ **E** Can sometimes lead to wrong conclusions

8 Which TWO of the following are true?

☐ **A** The annual prevalence of a condition reflects the number of new cases reported annually

☐ **B** Cohort studies are generally used to study a group of subjects with a particular disease and compare them with normal controls

☐ **C** In a frequency distribution, the mode is the most frequently observed value

☐ **D** If a measurement has a skewed distribution, then the mean and mode are always different

☐ **E** The standard deviation of a population may be smaller than the standard error of a sample mean from that population

9   **Choose THREE of these statements. The standard deviation of a group of observations**

☐ **A**   is the square of the variance of the group

☐ **B**   is a measure of the scatter of the observations around the mean

☐ **C**   is a valid statistical parameter only if the observations have a normal distribution

☐ **D**   is numerically higher than the standard error of the mean

☐ **E**   may be used as a basis for the calculation of the chi-squared value

10   **Which THREE of the following are correct statements about statistical items?**

☐ **A** $P = 0.01$ is a lower degree of statistical significance than $P = 0.05$

☐ **B**   The prevalence of ischaemic heart disease varies in different areas of the UK

☐ **C**   In a frequency distribution the mode is the most frequently observed value

☐ **D**   The median is the point on a scale of values which exactly divides the number of values into upper and lower halves

☐ **E**   The incidence of a disorder means the number suffering from that disorder at any one time

11 **The diastolic blood pressure readings of 1000 9-year-old children were found to have a statistically normal distribution with a mean value of 61 mmHg and a standard deviation of 8 mmHg. Which THREE of the following statements can be made about this study?**

- ☐ A The mean and standard deviation completely define the distribution of diastolic blood pressure for this age group

- ☐ B The mean diastolic blood pressure for this sample is equal to that of the whole population

- ☐ C 95% of the sample data lie within an interval defined by the mean ± 2 standard deviations (ie the range is 45–77 mmHg)

- ☐ D The median is 53 (ie 1 standard deviation below the mean)

- ☐ E The variance is 64 (ie the square of the standard deviation)

12 **A new antibiotic, Z, is compared with amoxicillin in a clinical trial. A higher proportion of those patients treated with Z respond in a given time (chi-squared value 4.2; $P = 0.05$). Which TWO of the following statements are true?**

- ☐ A The improved response to Z is clinically significant

- ☐ B Treatment with Z cannot be worse than treatment with amoxicillin

- ☐ C The results would be invalidated if there was a significant difference in the ages of the two treatment groups

- ☐ D The trial implies that a difference in response of 4.2 times was observed

- ☐ E The results may have occurred by chance 1 time in 20

13 In the clinical trial of a new treatment, which THREE statements apply?

☐ **A** The null hypothesis is true if there are significant differences between the response of the treatment and placebo groups

☐ **B** The patients should be randomised

☐ **C** Stratum matching of patients is necessary if the groups are small

☐ **D** In a type I error the null hypothesis is wrongly rejected

☐ **E** The number of subjects required decreases as the power of the trial increases

14 For the correlation coefficient r, which TWO of the following statements are correct?

☐ **A** The value of r lies between -1 and $+1$

☐ **B** If $r = 0.1$ this excludes a significant correlation between the variables

☐ **C** If r is negative, one value increases while the other decreases

☐ **D** r would be useful in comparing the relationship between blood pressure and cardiovascular mortality in a population

☐ **E** It can be used to predict one variable from the value of the other

15 **The time taken to walk 10 m was recorded in 50 patients who had suffered a stroke. The observations were found to be distributed symmetrically about the mean (47 s). Which THREE statements apply?**

☐ **A** The observations, being symmetrical about the mean, must follow a normal distribution

☐ **B** If the observations had been found to be positively skewed, their mode would have been less than the mean

☐ **C** The median time to walk 10 m is equal to the 50th percentile

☐ **D** Computing the variance of the observations would provide a measure of their spread about the mean

☐ **E** Computing the standard deviation of the observations would provide a measure of the reliability of the mean

16 **When looking at the referral rate to hospital specialists, which TWO of these are true?**

☐ **A** The greatest source of variation is the GP

☐ **B** Deprivation accounts for about one-third of the difference in referral rates

☐ **C** GP experience in a specialty decreases the rate of referral

☐ **D** Prescribing rate goes down as referral rate rises

☐ **E** The smallest referral rates are from the largest practices

17 **Select THREE of the following concerning a GP with 2000 patients over a 1-year period. A GP will see**

☐ **A** 21 cases of myocardial infarction

☐ **B** 12 cases of pneumonia

☐ **C** 32 cases of severe depression

☐ **D** 8 cases of new cancers

☐ **E** 6 patients with acute stroke

18 Select TWO items about the Oxcheck study

☐ **A** Looked at secondary prevention in coronary artery disease

☐ **B** Involved intensive, doctor-led intervention clinics in General Practice

☐ **C** Showed that clinics were expensive and the results of prevention strategy were disappointing

☐ **D** Moved focus to secondary prevention

SINGLE BEST ANSWER QUESTIONS

1   Select ONE option. In clinical governance:

☐ **A**   Doctor can choose whether to be involved in audit

☐ **B**   Good practice should be kept within the practice

☐ **C**   Leadership from the PCT should be sought

☐ **D**   Evidence-based medicine is a separate issue

☐ **E**   Risk management must be in place

2   Which ONE of these is NOT true? Clinical governance is concerned with

☐ **A**   Regulation by others

☐ **B**   Technical quality

☐ **C**   Risk management

☐ **D**   Efficiency

☐ **E**   Patient satisfaction

3   Which ONE of the following is most true of strokes?

☐ **A**   Are the commonest cause of disability in the UK

☐ **B**   Are the commonest cause of death in the UK

☐ **C**   About 20% of strokes are due to cerebral infarction

☐ **D**   Each stroke episode has a 5% mortality

☐ **E**   50% of strokes recur in the next year

4   A study finds that the height of a child compared with his or her siblings has values of $r = 0.6$, $P < 0.001$. Which ONE of the following is true?

☐ **A** r is the correlation coefficient of probability

☐ **B**   If $P < 0.001$ it means that the result is highly significant

☐ **C**   If $P < 0.001$ it means that too few measurements have been made

☐ **D**   If $r < 1$ then a negative correlation exists

☐ **E**   There is a definite linear relationship

5   Which ONE of these statements is NOT true in a normal (Gaussian) distribution?

☐ **A**   The mode is the most frequent observation

☐ **B**   The median divides the distribution exactly into two halves

☐ **C**   The mean, median and the mode are numerically the same

☐ **D**   The distribution is numerically the same as a Poisson distribution

☐ **E**   All the people in the sample are normal

6   The median is used in preference to the arithmetic mean when which ONE of these applies?

☐ **A**   The variance is large

☐ **B**   The sample size is small

☐ **C**   The observations are from a population with a skew distribution

☐ **D**   Observer error is likely to be large

☐ **E**   The chi-squared value is to be calculated

7 **An article in a medical journal states that in a study of gestational age at birth and neurological development at 12 months of age, r was found to be +0.56 and $P < 0.001$. Which statement is correct?**

☐ **A** r is the correlation coefficient of probability

☐ **B** There is a negative association between gestational age and neurological development

☐ **C** There is a significant relationship between gestational age and neurological development

☐ **D** Pre-term birth causes an inhibition in neurological development

☐ **E** The small value of P means that too few infants were studied

8 **In the UK, respiratory diseases account for which ONE of the following statements?**

☐ **A** A quarter of medical admissions

☐ **B** 1 in 10 deaths

☐ **C** 1 in 10 working days lost through illness

9 **Which ONE is the commonest diagnosis leading to wheelchair use in the UK?**

☐ **A** Arthritis

☐ **B** Cerebrovascular disease

☐ **C** Chronic obstructive pulmonary disease

☐ **D** Ischaemic heart disease

☐ **E** Amputation

☐ **F** Cancer

10 In intermittent claudication, which ONE of the following statements is NOT correct?

☐ **A** The clinical course is more benign in women than in men

☐ **B** Symptoms usually deteriorate steadily following presentation

☐ **C** Life expectancy is shorter than in unaffected individuals

☐ **D** Regular exercise improves blood flow in the long term

SUMMARY COMPLETION QUESION

THEME: BACK PAIN

In an attempt to improve the management of back pain in your practice you consider adopting the RCGP guidelines. The following paper describes a trial of the implementation of these guidelines. Read the extract and then the summary which critically appraises this trial. For each gap in the summary select the most appropriate term from the list below.

Implementation of RCGP guidelines for acute low back pain: a cluster randomised controlled trial. Dey *et al British Journal of General Practice* **2004;54:33–7**

Abstract

Background The Royal College of General Practitioners (RCGP) has produced guidelines for the management of acute low back pain in primary care.

Aim To investigate the impact on patient management of an educational strategy to promote these guidelines among general practitioners (GPs).

Design of study Group randomised controlled trial, using the health centre as the unit of randomisation.

Setting Primary care teams in north-west England.

Method Twenty-four health centres were randomly allocated to an intervention or control arm. Practices in the intervention arm were offered outreach visits to promote national guidelines on acute low back pain, as well as access to fast-track physiotherapy and to a triage service for patients with persistent symptoms.

Results Twenty-four centres were randomised. Two thousand, one hundred and eighty-seven eligible patients presented with acute low back pain during the study period: 1049 in the intervention group and 1138 in the control group. There were no significant differences between the study groups in the proportion of patients who were referred for X-ray, issued with a sickness certificate, prescribed opioids or muscle relaxants, or who were referred to secondary care, but significantly more patients in the intervention group were referred to physiotherapy or the back pain unit (difference in proportion = 12.2%, 95% confidence interval (CI) = 2.8% to 21.6%).

Conclusion The management of patients presenting with low back pain to primary care was mostly unchanged by an outreach educational strategy to promote greater adherence to RCGP guidelines among GPs. An increase in referral to physiotherapy or educational programmes followed the provision of a triage service.

Summary

Guidelines are everywhere, but what makes a guideline successful? It must be clinically relevant and simple to follow, but ultimately a guideline is only successful if people use it. A good candidate for a successful guideline is acute back pain: it is a common condition, simple triage systems exist and effective treatment may improve long term outcomes. This paper examines the impact of an educational strategy to promote the use of a guideline on patient management. A____**(1)**____is an appropriate tool to investigate the impact of the educational strategy____**(2)**____on clinical management____**(3)**____, but this study will not provide any data on the impact on symptoms. The study does not look at____**(4)**____outcomes such as certified time off work or duration of symptoms, but rather changes in management, eg use of X-ray.

The authors aim to assess the impact of the educational strategy on management, but the intervention is not restricted to the educational sessions. The intervention groups differ from the control group not only in the fact that they have had the educational input, but also in the fact that they have access to a fast-track physio clinic and triage service. No steps have been taken to____**(5)**____the influence of the added resources on management. Are the____**(6)**____practices managing back pain to the best of their abilities within the limited resources available? Would the provision of these resources change behaviour regardless of any educational input or guidelines? The confounding influence of the extra resources must be accounted for when examining the effect of the intervention.

The results of this study are____(7)____, there is no evidence of changes in management with the exception of referrals to physio or back clinic. Although the randomised control trial is methodologically appropriate, the design does not allow us to quantify the impact of the intervention on individual practices. More insight might have been gained had the authors looked at management before and after the intervention. This study____(8)____support the use of an educational strategy to promote guidelines.

Options

A   Quantify

B   Inconclusive

C   Intervention

D   Clinical

E   Qualify

F   Randomised controlled trial

G   Remove

H   Does

I   Outcome

J   Control

K   Does not

L   Double blind RCT

M   Insignificant

N   Surrogate

O   Significant

SUMMARY COMPLETION QUESTION

THEME: COX-2 INHIBITORS

You practice in an area with a large elderly population. One of your partners has recently attended a meeting sponsored by a drug company at which data were presented that apparently show COX-2 inhibitors to be superior in side-effect profile to conventional NSAIDs. He suggests the practice adopt these drugs as first-line anti-inflammatories in the elderly. Read the extract from the results section of the paper below, followed by the critique. For each gap in the critique, select the most appropriate response from the list of options.

Observational study of upper gastrointestinal haemorrhage in elderly patients given selective cyclo-oxygenase-2 inhibitors or conventional non-steroidal anti-inflammatory drugs. Mamdani *et al British Medical Journal* 2002;325:624–7

Methods

Study design We conducted a population based retrospective cohort study by linking administrative healthcare databases covering over 1.3 million patients aged 66 years or more in Ontario, Canada, from 17 April 2000 through to 31 March 2001. Ontario's elderly population has universal access to prescription drugs, hospital care and doctor services. This study was approved by the Ethics Review Board of Sunnybrook and Women's College Health Sciences Centre.

Cohort definition We compared users of rofecoxib, celecoxib, non-selective NSAIDs, or the combination of diclofenac plus misoprostol with a random sample of 100, 000 controls dispensed none of these drugs. Despite the potential differences in morbidity between users of NSAIDs and non-users, we chose patients not using NSAIDs as the control group for two reasons: firstly, such a control group provides useful baseline risk estimates of upper gastrointestinal haemorrhage not related to NSAID use, and, secondly, most previous studies of the association between NSAID use and upper gastrointestinal haemorrhage have non-users of NSAIDs as controls. Thus, choosing non-users of NSAIDs as our control group allowed comparison of our incidence and relative risk estimates with such studies. We also conducted pairwise comparisons of the different NSAID study groups in relation to each other.

For the four drug cohorts, the first NSAID prescription during the study period after a patient's 66th birthday served as the index date. To create a cohort of NSAID-naive subjects within these four drug groups, we excluded individuals who were dispensed an NSAID in the year preceding the index date. We also excluded subjects given NSAIDs from more than one of the study's four groups of drug on the same day. To exclude sporadic users of NSAIDs, we included only those individuals who were given at least two successive prescriptions of NSAID and who received enough drug for at least 30 days of observation. Events occurring during this initial 30-day period were included in the analysis.

To create the control cohort, all Ontario residents not included in any of the above cohorts were randomly assigned index dates from 17 April 2000 to 15 March 2001, as in the drug cohorts. Individuals aged 66 years and older who were alive on the assigned index date were screened for NSAID use. From those without a prescription for any NSAID in the year before the index date or during the observation period, we randomly selected 100, 000 individuals to form the control cohort. This group was not matched for age or sex to any of the drug cohorts, but represented the general elderly population of Ontario not prescribed NSAIDs.

We repeated the analyses using controls matched by age (within one year of the birth date) and sex to all patients in the four drug cohorts as a sensitivity analysis. Because women are more likely than men to receive NSAIDs and may have a lower risk for upper gastrointestinal haemorrhage, we repeated the analyses separately for men and women. Finally, we repeated the upper gastrointestinal haemorrhage analysis after excluding subjects with a history of such bleeds.

| | Study cohort | | | | |
	Community controls	Non-selective NSAIDs	Diclofenac + misoprostol	Rofecoxib	Celecoxib
No of patients (% women)	(n = 100 000) 100 000 (55)	(n = 5391) 5 391 (59)	(n = 5087) 5 087 (62)	(n = 14 583) 14 583 (72)	(n = 18 908) 18 908 (70)
Mean (SD) age (years)	75.4 (7.3)	75.5 (7.0)	76.6 (7.1)	76.5 (6.9)	76.5 (6.8)
Residence in long-term care facility	4 074 (4)	398 (7)	503 (10)	652 (4)	810 (4)
Low income status	21 073 (21)	1 831 (34)	1 725 (34)	4 445 (30)	5 673 (30)
Hospitalisation in past year	11 513 (12)	1 023 (19)	925 (18)	2 900 (20)	3 651 (19)
Mean (SD) no of prescription drugs in past year	5.4 (5.4)	8.3 (6.4)	8.3 (6.4)	9.9 (6.5)	9.5 (6.4)
Use of gastroprotective agents within 180 days before entry to cohort	17 279 (17)	1 329 (25)	1 265 (25)	6 140 (42)	7 738 (41)
Use of narcotic analgesics within 180 days before entry to cohort	10 623 (11)	1 419 (26)	1 321 (26)	4 511 (31)	5 587 (30)

Hospitalisations or procedures in past 5 years:					
Malignancy	4 785 (5)	371 (7)	294 (6)	760 (5)	1 004 (5)
Prior upper gastrointestinal haemorrhage	1 440 (1)	64 (1)	66 (1)	369 (3)	476 (3)
Prior gastrointestinal or radiological procedure	17 839 (18)	1 090 (20)	1 043 (21)	4 731 (32)	5 855 (31)
Drug use in 120 days before index date to end of follow up:					
Aspirin	11 564 (12)	1 014 (19)	945 (19)	2 629 (18)	3 311 (18)
Anticoagulants	6 716 (7)	244 (5)	266 (5)	1 515 (10)	1 929 (10)
Antihyperglycaemics	9 256 (9)	756 (14)	706 (14)	1 819 (12)	2 344 (12)
Antirheumatics	0	66 (1)	71 (1)	401 (3)	865 (5)
Glucocorticoids	3 789 (4)	458 (9)	384 (8)	1 928 (13)	2 471 (13)
Gastroprotective agents:	16 394 (16)	1 699 (32)	1 277 (25)	6 213 (43)	7 793 (41)
Proton pump inhibitors	6 139 (6)	432 (8)	405 (8)	3 156 (22)	3 868 (20)
Other*	11 615 (12)	1 407 (26)	983 (19)	3 754 (26)	4 778 (25)

*Includes histamine-H_2 receptor antagonists, misoprostol, and sucralfate.

Table 1 Characteristics of cohorts in study of elderly patients using different NSAIDs. Values are numbers (percentages) unless stated otherwise

		Study cohort			
	Community controls (n=100 000)	Non-selective NSAIDs (n=5391)	Diclofenac + misoprostol (n=5087)	Rofecoxib (n=14 583)	Celecoxib (n=18 908)
No of admissions for upper gastrointestinal haemorrhage	82	17	13	43	32
Mean (SD) days of follow up	138.7 (77.4)	91.7 (68.3)	97.8 (71.2)	146.9 (89.6)	170.3 (97.0)
Total follow up (person years)	37 981	1353	1361	5865	8818
No of upper gastrointestinal haemorrhages per 1000 person years	2.2	12.6	9.6	7.3	3.6
Model based risk ratios (95% CI):					
Unadjusted	1.0 (reference)	6.1 (3.6 to 10.2)	4.6 (2.5 to 8.2)	3.5 (2.4 to 5.0)	1.7 (1.1 to 2.6)
Adjusted	1.0 (reference)	4.0 (2.3 to 6.9)	3.0 (1.7 to 5.5)	1.9 (1.3 to 2.8)	1.0 (0.7 to 1.6)
Number needed to treat to harm (NNT(H))*	N/A	403	592	1389	N/A

* NNT(H) calculations are based on a follow up of 295 days from the Cox proportional hazard model estimates.

Table 2. Upper gastrointestinal haemorrhage among elderly patients using different NSAIDs

Critique

Studies of this nature are fraught with difficulty and are awash with potential confounding influences. The elderly population of most Western economies is extremely diverse, with the effects of a lifetime of lifestyle, genetic and medical influences becoming more evident with time. Comparison of different socioeconomic groups reveals large variation in morbidity and mortality and this must be accounted for in comparing____(1)____. The authors set out to collect prescription data and compared this with gastrointestinal outcomes. The control group was not matched to any of the intervention cohorts, but reflected the general elderly population.

This approach while pragmatic, leaves the results at the mercy of the biggest confounder of all: general health. While the study does attempt to accommodate some confounding influences, including low income, retrospective hospital admission and prescription drug use, inclusion of a well-being indicator would allow more accurate comparison. No attempt is made to control for tobacco or alcohol use. Furthermore, the study does not collect data on____(2)____outcomes after initiation of COX-2s. There is increasing evidence of excess____(3)____mortality with COX-2s, possibly through differential effects on platelets. If we are looking for evidence of superior side-effect profiles,____(4)____morbidity and mortality should be considered.

The study design does not account for OTC use of NSAIDs, and does not attempt to ____(5)____ the patients according to indication for COX-2 rather than conventional NSAID. Patients were excluded if they had taken an NSAID in the year before the study. It may be that patients given COX-2s had previously had side-effects from NSAIDs prescribed over one year ago or had a previous history of dyspepsia, as suggested from the significantly higher use of____(6)____in the COX-2 cohorts. Indeed, this represents one of the biggest differences between the groups, and also one of the most potent confounders when looking at the outcome of upper GI haemorrhage.

The results in Table 2 suggest significant increase in risk among NSAID users compared to COX-2 users in the ___**(7)**___ data. ___**(8)**___ data show no increase for celecoxib and double the risk for rofecoxib, however, the 95% confidence intervals approach 1. The NNT(H) is ___**(9)**___ for ___**(10)**___ than ___**(11)**___ cohorts, implying many more people need to take these drugs for one ___**(12)**___ outcome.

Options

A   NSAID

B   Adverse

C   Gastroprotective agents

D   Controls

E   Stratify

F   Gastrointestinal

G   Antacids

H   Cohorts

I   Unadjusted

J   Selective

K   Overall

L   Non-gastrointestinal

M   Increased

N   Higher

O   Beneficial

P   Adjusted

R   Cardiovascular

S   Lower

T   Rofecoxib

U   Celecoxib

V   Anticoagulant

MEDICINE ANSWERS

CARDIOVASCULAR

EXTENDED MATCHING QUESTIONS

THEME: PULSES

1	D	Plateau
2	E	Pulsus alternans
3	C	Collapsing
4	B	Bisferiens
5	E	Pulsus alternans
6	F	Pulsus paradoxus
7	F	Pulsus paradoxus
8	D	Plateau

Plateau pulse is found in aortic stenosis, it is of low amplitude and has a slow rise and fall. Collapsing or waterhammer pulse is found in aortic regurgitation. Pulsus alternans is found in left ventricular failure, there are alternate large- and small-amplitude beats, and it is usually found when taking blood pressure. An apparent doubling in rate is noted as the mercury level falls.

Bisferiens is a double-topped pulse, found in mixed aortic stenosis and regurgitation. Pulsus paradoxus is found in cardiac tamponade and severe COPD and the volume decreases markedly with inspiration.

THEME: ECG FINDINGS

9 **H** Short PR interval

10 **A** Absent P waves with ragged baseline

11 **F** Peaked T wave

12 **C** Large R waves in V1–V2

13 **I** Short QT interval

14 **G** Prolonged PR interval

15 **B** Inverted T wave

16 **E** Long QT interval

17 **D** Large S waves in V1–V2

ECG changes can be important and you will need to be aware of them. Right ventricular hypertrophy can result in large R waves in V1–V2 and large S waves in V5–V6. Similarly, left ventricular hypertrophy can result in large R waves in V5–V6 and large S waves in V1–V2. The PR interval is lengthened in first-degree heart block and shortened in Wolff–Parkinson–White syndrome. Atrial fibrillation will show absent P waves on a ragged baseline. T waves will be peaked in hyperkalaemia, and inverted in bundle branch block, ischaemia and ventricular hypertrophy. The QT interval will be lengthened in hypocalcaemia and shortened in hypercalcaemia.

MULTIPLE BEST ANSWER QUESTIONS

1   Mediterranean diet   Answers: B C

A Mediterranean diet consists of fruit, fish, vegetables and poultry. It appears to decrease coronary artery disease more than the reduction achieved by a low-fat diet.

2   Exercise   Answers: A C D E

Regular exercise lowers blood pressure, and decreases the risk of cancer of the colon, depression and diabetes. Co-ordination is improved and the elderly may particularly benefit.

3   Myocardial infarction   Answers: A C D

Following myocardial infarction (MI) ventricular fibrillation is most likely to occur within the first few hours and is one of the more easily correctable causes of early death. The ECG can remain normal following even an extensive MI. Thrombolytic therapy, when indicated, should be started early and is not dependent on resolution of chest pain.

4   Angina pectoris   Answers: A E

Angina with normal coronary arteries is found in cardiomyopathies, severe aortic stenosis and pulmonary hypertension, as well as in otherwise normal hearts when coronary artery spasm or coronary blood flow abnormalities are implicated. The resting ECG is normal in 50% or more of patients between attacks. Many patients have angina on getting up in the morning and become symptom-free later in the day. ST segment elevation during an attack is unusual but may occur in 'variant' angina. The mechanism of angina on lying down is unknown but this symptom usually indicates severe coronary disease.

5   Deep venous thrombosis   Answers: B C D

The most common cause of DVT is major surgery, especially after the age of 40. Long-distance travel does cause DVT and several cases have been reported. It is best to stop the combined contraceptive pill four weeks before major surgery. Calf vein thrombosis can be treated using compression bandages alone. Varicose veins have been shown to be a risk factor.

SINGLE BEST ANSWER QUESTIONS

1   Isolated systolic hypertension in the elderly   **Answer: C**

Isolated systolic hypertension in the elderly affects about 50% of people over 60. It confers no significant cardiovascular risk, and it is important to treat isolated systolic hypertension. Pulse pressure is a better predictor of risk than diastolic or systolic blood pressure.

2   British Hypertension Society Guidelines   **Answer: D**

British Hypertension Society Guidelines recommend that adults should have their blood pressure checked every five years, suggest that drug treatment is of proven value until the age of 80 years, and advise that non-pharmacological advice should be offered to all patients. Drug treatment should be tailored to the patient; the resource implications for GPs are massive.

3   Atrial fibrillation   **Answer: C**

Atrial fibrillation (AF) is associated with a substantial increase in the risk of stroke, and the risk associated with AF increases with age. Patients have considerable concerns about taking warfarin. In AF, rate control is as important as rhythm control.

4   Mortality rate following myocardial infarction   **Answer: A**

Age is an important factor in deciding the outcome of an infarct. Low blood pressure is a poor prognostic feature in the post-infarction phase. High heart rate on admission to hospital, anterior infarction pattern on ECG and previous myocardial infarction are poor prognostic indicators.

5   Angioplasty   **Answer: E**

The main stem of the left coronary artery is not suitable for angioplasty because occlusion during attempted angioplasty might be catastrophic. Multiple vessel angioplasty is now commonplace. Previous bypass surgery is not a contraindication to angioplasty, which may offer fewer risks than repeat surgery. The treatment of unstable angina may account for 25–30% of procedures in some centres.

PHOTO QUESTION

THEME: CARDIOLOGY

1   ECG 1 B   Diagnosis: Inferior MI

The history is suggestive of ischaemic heart disease both in the symptoms described and the previous history. The ECG shows typical ST changes in leads II, III and aVF. The lateral leads also show signs of ischaemia.

2   ECG 2 A   Diagnosis: Pericarditis

This patient is complaining of typical symptoms of pericarditis, and examination may reveal a pericardial rub at the apex. The ECG shows typical changes in the ST segments, which are often described as concave upwards, rather than convex upwards as seen in ischaemia.

3   ECG 3 D   Diagnosis: Ventricular tachycardia

The ECG shows a broad complex tachycardia, characteristic of VT.

4   ECG 4 E   Diagnosis: Second-degree AV block
(Wenckebach block)

The ECG shows increasing PR interval until conduction fails and the P wave is not followed by a QRS complex. It is relatively common after inferior MI when the infarction affects the conducting system. Treatment is seldom necessary.

5   ECG 5 C   Diagnosis: Atrial flutter

Atrial flutter is associated with rheumatic heart disease, ischaemic and hypertensive disease. Normal QRS complexes are seen with sawtooth appearance of the atrial activity. Atrial rate is usually around 300, with 2:1, 3:1 or 4:1 block.

DERMATOLOGY/ENT/ OPHTHALMOLOGY

DERMATOLOGY

EXTENDED MATCHING QUESTIONS

THEME: RASHES

1	A	Dermatitis artefacta
2	C	Lichen simplex
3	B	Dermatitis herpetiformis
4	D	Nodular prurigo

Suspect dermatitis artefacta if there are straight edges to the rash. Lichen simplex will heal if scratching is stopped. Nodular prurigo is one cause of rash on the hands.

THEME: CAUSES OF NAIL DISCOLORATION

5	F	Yellow nail syndrome
6	C	Penicillamine
7	A	Chloroquine
8	B	Leuconychia
9	E	Trauma
10	D	Tinea infection
11	B	Leuconychia

Penicillamine may stain the nails yellow, whereas chloroquine may stain the nails a blue-grey colour. Following trauma, often of a minor nature, the nails often have white streaks. Leuconychia is said to be inherited as an autosomal dominant disorder; the whole nail becomes

white. Tineal infection can cause yellow thickened areas of the nails
with slow growth. In yellow nail syndrome the nail is curved
longitudinally and transversely; there is an association with
lymphoedema.

THEME: RASHES

12 C   Infected eczema

13 B   Ichthyosis

14 A   Erythema multiforme

15 D   Pustular psoriasis

16 E   Scabies

With scabies, you will need to look carefully for burrows on the sides
of the fingers. The lesions of pustular psoriasis are often seen on the
soles of the feet and palms of the hands. Ichthyosis will cause scaly dry
skin on the fingers. Erythema multiforme characteristically is seen as a
large vesicle with a surrounding red halo. Infected eczema often has
secondary staphylococcal infection.

THEME: LEG ULCERS

17 B   Venous ulcers

18 B   Venous ulcers

19 A   Ischaemic ulcers

20 A   Ischaemic ulcers

21 B   Venous ulcers

It is important to be able to distinguish between venous and arterial leg
ulcers. Venous ulcers are painless and pigmented, and there is usually
oedema and induration with eczematous skin surrounding the ulcer.
Ischaemic leg ulcers tend to be punched out and necrotic; they are
frequently painful.

THEME: SKIN CONDITIONS

22 E Guttate psoriasis

23 F Irritant contact dermatitis

24 H Pompholyx

25 D Erythrodermic psoriasis

26 B Asteatotic eczema

Irritant contact dermatitis differs from allergic contact dermatitis in that the area affected corresponds to the area of exposure. Allergic contact dermatitis tends to be progressively severe with repeated exposure and may cause irritation at distant sites, eg the dermatitis is caused by earrings and watches in the case of nickel sensitivity. Psoriasis is generally diagnosable by its characteristic lesions, which show pinpoint bleeding when removed.

MULTIPLE BEST ANSWER QUESTIONS

1   Nails   Answers: A B C

Decreased nutritional supply to the nail matrix can lead to defective nail formation, resulting in a transverse groove made of thinner nail plate. Since fingernails grow at about 1 mm/week it is possible to date previous illnesses. The other major cause of these grooves is psoriasis. Opacity of the nail is suggestive of diabetes mellitus, cardiac failure and psoriasis. Blue nails are found as a side-effect of antimalarial drugs such as chloroquine; green nails are caused by *Pseudomonas* spp. Splinter haemorrhages are seen in bacterial endocarditis. Longitudinal ridges can be seen in lichen planus.

2   Pregnancy   Answers: B D

The condition of most patients with atopic eczema improves during pregnancy. However, some patients suffer deterioration which may be caused by increased excoriation from pruritus gravidarum. Hidradenitis suppurativa also usually improves during pregnancy.

3   Drug reactions   Answers: B E

Oral contraceptives are characteristically linked with melasma, a brownish pigmentation on the face. Both codeine and aspirin can cause urticaria. Exfoliative dermatitis is usually caused by carbamazepine, allopurinol, gold, phenytoin, captopril or diltiazem but not tetracycline. Fucidin® usually causes eczema rather than pigmentation.

4   Granuloma annulare   Answers: C D E

Granuloma annulare is a disease of unknown aetiology which often starts in a single area but may develop into multiple lesions. It is usually confined to the extremities and is painless. The disease may persist for many years and there is no effective treatment. There is a probable association with diabetes mellitus.

5 Erythema nodosum   Answers: B C

Herpes simplex is usually associated with erythema multiforme.
Hyperthyroidism usually causes pruritus or urticaria rather than
erythema nodosum. The infections associated with erythema nodosum
include tuberculosis and leprosy. Inflammatory bowel disease and many
rheumatic diseases are associated with erythema nodosum.

6 Drugs that exacerbate psoriasis   Answers: A D

Lithium and beta-blockers can precipitate and exacerbate psoriasis.
Hydralazine has been linked with a number of conditions, for example
systemic lupus erythematosus, but not psoriasis.

7 Alopecia areata   Answers: B D E

Hair loss in alopecia areata may occur at any site. Most of the follicles
retain the ability to form new hairs. Alopecia areata may be associated
with frank or subclinical autoimmune thyroid disease and with Down's
syndrome. Nail pitting or roughness is commonly found in alopecia
areata.

8 Acne vulgaris   Answers: A B C

In 60% of teenagers acne will be of sufficient severity for them to treat
themselves with proprietary preparations or seek medical advice.
Circulating levels of androgen are usually normal in patients with acne.
The blackhead is caused by the plug within the pilosebaceous duct
expanding to dilate the pilosebaceous orifice and gradually become
extruded. The severity of acne is directly related to the degree of
secretion of sebum.

SINGLE BEST ANSWER QUESTIONS

1   Basal cell carcinoma   **Answer: A**

Basal cell carcinoma (BCC) is the most common skin malignancy in Caucasians. Basal cell carcinoma sometimes occurs on covered skin sites. Curettage and cautery in skilled hands remains a perfectly acceptable means of treatment.

2   Multiple seborrhoeic warts   **Answer: A**

Seborrhoeic warts may occur in any area where there are pilosebaceous follicles, but they are seen predominantly on the face and trunk. They are non-infective. They are best removed by curettage or cryotherapy.

3   Erythema nodosum   **Answer: A**

Erythema nodosum may be due to an underlying systemic disease, eg Crohn's disease, ulcerative colitis or sarcoidosis. It can be caused by various drugs, notably sulphonamides and oral contraceptives, and by preceding infection, especially streptococcal.

4   Molluscum contagiosum   **Answer: A**

A review in the *BMJ* in 1999 found that scarring was most common after phenol ablation. Furthermore there was no evidence to support any of the treatments over watchful waiting. The condition is most commonly seen in children but is also seen in HIV-positive patients. The average duration of the condition is eight months.

5   Venous leg ulcers   **Answer: B**

Only compression bandaging has been shown to be effective. Hyperbaric oxygen is a treatment for radio-osteonecrosis. The key to safe and effective treatment of venous ulcers is measurement of the ankle:brachial blood pressure index to avoid inadvertent treatment of arterial ulcers.

PHOTO QUESTION

THEME: DERMATOLOGY

1   C   Diagnosis: Varicose eczema

Chronic venous hypertension as a result of varicose veins results in extravasation and haemosiderin deposition particularly around the ankles. Successful control requires support hosiery.

2   A   Diagnosis: Psoriasis

This image shows the characteristic lesions of psoriasis. Stable plaque psoriasis should not routinely be treated with steroids, rather emollients, coal tar preparations or vitamin D analogues are the treatment of choice. Many patients report that their psoriasis improves on their summer holidays.

3   B   Diagnosis: Neurofibromatosis

An autosomal dominant pattern of inheritance, patients typically have neurofibromas, café au lait patches and may be associated with acoustic neuromas, gliomas and phaeochromocytomas.

4   E   Diagnosis: Phototoxicity

This resembles sunburn rather than eczema, and is characteristically seen in sun exposed areas. It may be caused by dyes, plants and drugs including thiazides, sulphonamides and amiodarone.

5   D   Diagnosis: Fire coral

Photo of wrist. This shows a characteristic local toxic reaction to a stinging hydroid, in this case coral. These usually settle spontaneously, but topical steroids may be necessary for severe irritation.

ENT

EXTENDED MATCHING QUESTIONS

THEME: LESIONS ON THE EAR

1	A	Chilblains
2	E	Squamous cell cancer
3	F	Tophi
4	B	Kerato-acanthoma
5	D	Rodent ulcer
6	C	Psoriatic

Chilblains are common, painful and itchy. Squamous cell cancer lesions of the ear are slow-growing lesions found on the helix. Tophi in the ear are usually found on the antihelix. Kerato-acanthoma lesions are rapidly growing and are also usually found on the helix. Rodent ulcer ear lesions are usually found behind and below the ear. Psoriatic lesions are found in the external auditory meatus and on the skin behind and below the ear.

THEME: HOARSENESS

7	D	Pharyngeal neoplasia
8	E	Smoking
9	C	Myxoedema
10	D	Pharyngeal neoplasia
11	B	Gastro-oesophageal reflux

Hoarseness is an abnormality of the voice. If associated with weight loss, consider upper or lower respiratory tract cancer. Smoking causes trauma to the larynx. Associated dysphagia is suggestive of upper respiratory cancer and palsies of the larynx or pharynx. Long-standing myxoedema is associated with a hoarse voice.

THEME: EARACHE

12 I   Ramsay Hunt syndrome

13 D   Glue ear

14 J   Cerebellopontine angle tumours

15 A   Otitis media

16 B   Otitis externa

Ramsay Hunt syndrome, herpes zoster oticus, is treated with aciclovir. It may be associated with facial nerve palsy. Acoustic neuromas may be misdiagnosed as Ménière's and should be suspected, particularly in patients with unilateral sensorineural deafness. Viral otitis media commonly causes a febrile illness in children with few localising symptoms. Examination should always include the ears, nose and throat. Otitis externa may be secondary to minor ear trauma, middle ear disease or caused by repeated immersion, eg in surfers and swimmers.

MULTIPLE BEST ANSWER QUESTIONS

1   Glue ear   **Answers: A E**

Atopic children have increased incidence and episodes tend to be more
prolonged. Bottle-fed babies have greater incidence of atopy. Children
with facial anomalies are more prone to glue ear due to poor drainage.
Neomycin and meningitis cause sensorineural deafness.

2   Oral cancer   **Answers: A B E**

Several studies have shown an association between high alcohol
consumption and oral cancer. Iron deficiency, but not folate deficiency,
predisposes to oral cancer. Cigar smoking is associated with leukoplakia
of the floor of the mouth in women.

3   Otitis externa   **Answers: A C D**

Any local trauma (eg poking the ears, foreign body in the ear) will
predispose to otitis externa. Certain occupations, such as mining and
diving, have an increased incidence of otitis externa. Usually, otitis
media is more common in the under fives. Psoriasis, eczema and
seborrhoeic dermatitis are predisposing factors.

4   Drugs causing dry mouth   **Answers: B D E**

Antihistamines, phenothiazines and amphetamines can cause a dry
mouth. Tricyclic, but not monoamine oxidase inhibitor, antidepressants
cause a dry mouth, as do bronchodilators but bronchoconstrictors do
not.

SINGLE BEST ANSWER QUESTIONS

1   Conductive deafness   **Answer: A**

Post-meningitis, congenital rubella and kernicterus cause sensorineural deafness rather than conductive deafness, which is caused by glue ear, large perforations, and destructions, dislocation or adhesion of the ossicles.

2   Mild allergic rhinitis   **Answer: B**

The best initial treatment for mild allergic rhinitis is an oral non-sedating antihistamine. Chronic nasal blockage may require the use of nasal steroids. Regular use of xylometazoline may cause rhinitis medicamentosa, a paradoxical increase in rhinitis. RAST testing is unnecessary unless a specific trigger is suspected or symptoms are particularly severe. Reduction in house dust mite exposure has not been shown to significantly reduce symptoms.

3   Sensorineural deafness   **Answer: D**

The commonest cause of isolated sensorineural deafness in this age group is presbyacusis. In Ménière's disease, symptoms of tinnitus, vertigo and a fullness are common. Infections such as measles and mumps, or ototoxic medications would usually present earlier. Barotrauma and otosclerosis are causes of conductive deafness.

PHOTO QUESTION

THEME: AUDIOGRAMS

1   A   Diagnosis: Noise-induced hearing loss

The audiogram shows bilateral high frequency loss, typical of noise damage.

2   B   Diagnosis: Presbyacusis

This audiogram shows moderate loss in the higher frequencies, often seen in older patients who may complain that everyday noises such as speech sound flat.

3   C   Diagnosis: Normal

4   D   Diagnosis: Severe bilateral hearing loss

This audiogram shows severe loss over a large range of frequencies and is likely to require hearing aids.

5   E   Diagnosis: Severe unilateral hearing loss

Once causes of conductive hearing loss are excluded, unilateral hearing loss requires investigation to exclude nerve lesions.

OPHTHALMOLOGY

EXTENDED MATCHING QUESTIONS

THEME: SUDDEN LOSS OF VISION

1   **C**   Optic neuritis

2   **D**   Senile macular degeneration

3   **E**   Toxic optic neuropathy

4   **B**   Migraine

5   **A**   Central retinal vein occlusion

In the sudden loss of vision associated with migraine, there is a complete recovery from the loss of vision which often, but not always, occurs with headache. In central retinal vein occlusion, the visual loss develops over a few hours. There is extensive haemorrhage visible in the fundus.

Senile macular degeneration is a gradually progressive loss of vision in an older person. There is preservation of peripheral fields. Optic neuritis is a gradual loss of vision, usually occurring in people between 20 and 45 years old. The peripheral vision is intact. Toxic optic neuropathy tends to occur in heavy cigarette smokers. Peripheral vision remains largely intact.

THEME: RED EYE

6 **D**   Keratitis

7 **B**   Episcleritis

8 **C**   Iritis

9 **A**   Acute glaucoma

10 **E**   Subconjunctival haemorrhage

In the red eye caused by episcleritis, there is slight or no pain. Vision tends to be normal and the red eye will settle without treatment. Subconjunctival haemorrhage is painless and vision is normal. Keratitis is associated with impaired vision. An ulcer may be found near the visual axis. Acute glaucoma is accompanied by severe pain with severe visual impairment. Vomiting commonly occurs. In iritis, the pupil is small and often distorted.

THEME: VISUAL FIELD DEFECTS

11 **A**   Arcuate scotoma

12 **C**   Centrocaecal scotoma

13 **D**   Ring scotoma

14 **B**   Central scotoma

Visual field defects can be important in localising and defining a disease process. A central scotoma is characteristic of disease affecting the macula, whereas toxic neuropathy can produce a centrocaecal scotoma. A ring scotoma is the typical field defect in retinitis pigmentosa, while an arcuate scotoma is characteristic of glaucoma.

THEME: EYE LESIONS

15 D   Pterygium

16 A   Corneal arcus

17 E   Subconjunctival haemorrhage

18 B   Kayser–Fleischer rings

19 C   Pinguecula

20 B   Kayser–Fleischer rings

21 E   Subconjunctival haemorrhage

Pingueculae and pterygia are both found between the canthus and the corneal edge. A pterygium is a triangular fold of conjunctiva, whereas a pinguecula is a yellow deposit beneath the conjunctiva. A corneal arcus is very common and is a white ring near the outer margin of the cornea. Kayser–Fleischer rings are very rare, occurring in Wilson's disease as a deposit of copper at the periphery of the cornea. Subconjunctival haemorrhages are very common. They are bright red marks arising spontaneously or from prolonged forceful coughing or straining.

MULTIPLE BEST ANSWER QUESTIONS

1   Acute iritis   Answers: B C

Acute iritis causes blurred vision with photophobia and a small pupil. Needs to be referred at once as it is a threat to sight. Purulent discharge usually signifies conjunctivitis, while a hard and tender eye suggests acute glaucoma.

2   Ophthalmoscopy in myopia   Answers: A D

When conducting ophthalmoscopy in a patient with myopia, the minus lenses will be needed. The disc may look large and pale and there may be surrounding chorioretinal atrophy.

3   Ocular fundus findings   Answers: B D F G

Hard exudates are caused by lipoprotein leaking out of blood vessels and are noted in diabetes and hypertension. They are well-defined yellow-white deposits, often in rings. Soft exudates look like deposits of cotton wool. They occur in infarcted retina, often being associated with features of retinal ischaemia such as new vessel formation and venous dilatation. Soft exudates are due to the swelling of the axons in the nerve fibre layer of the retina.

SINGLE BEST ANSWER QUESTIONS

1   Causes of blindness   **Answer: D**

Macular degeneration accounts for over one-third of those blind over
the age of 65 years.

2   Causes of blindness   **Answer: A**

Diabetic retinopathy causes about 20% of the blindness in patients in
the age range 45–64 years.

3   Cataracts   **Answer: B**

In many cases, cataracts are age-related, appearing first when a person
is in his or her 40s or 50s, but not affecting vision until after age 60.
Other causes of cataracts include injury to the eye, untreated eye
inflammation, diabetes, drugs (such as cortisone), exposure to X-rays
and ultraviolet (UV) light, and heredity. Congenital cataracts may occur
as a result of an infection that happened during pregnancy, especially
toxoplasmosis, cytomegalovirus, syphilis, rubella or herpes simplex. In
infants and young children, cataracts may also be one symptom of a
metabolic disease affecting the body's processing of carbohydrates,
amino acids, calcium or copper. Myotonic dystrophy is associated with
early cataracts.

4   Diabetic maculopathy   **Answer: A**

Maculopathy as opposed to retinopathy is certainly more common in
the older patient with NIDDM. The patient may be registered blind
because of the damage to the very sensitive macular area. However,
even though the patient may be unable to read, they may retain
excellent peripheral vision. Treatment of maculopathy is usually with
small, focal laser burns to the macular area, avoiding the fovea. This is
in contrast to treatment for proliferative retinopathy which usually
involves several thousand burns to the peripheral retina. Drusen are a
normal feature in some patients. Hard exudates, often in rings, are
characteristic of diabetic maculopathy. Painful visual loss is not a
feature of maculopathy and would suggest glaucoma, uveitis or another
lesion.

5   Anterior uveitis   **Answer: B**

Blurring of vision, small pupil and photophobia suggest anterior uveitis. Other causes of 'red eye' are subconjunctival haemorrhage, which is not painful, and acute closed-angle glaucoma and keratitis, which are painful.

PHOTO QUESTION

THEME: OPHTHALMOLOGY

1   C   **Diagnosis: Anterior ischaemic optic neuropathy (AION)**

Symptoms of temporal arteritis require prompt action to avoid the other eye being affected. Typical features include age >60 years old, temporal headache, jaw claudication, systemic upset and raised ESR. The retina shows a swollen and pale optic nerve (due to infarction). A unilateral pale swollen disc is always AION. Where this is bilateral, it may be caused by papilloedema.

2   E   **Diagnosis: Normal**

This patient's symptoms are unrelated to his eyes.

3   A   **Diagnosis: Diabetic retinopathy**

The photo shows scattered blot haemorrhages, hard exudates and microaneuryms. These changes are the result of microangiopathic damage resulting in leakage of blood, lipoprotein and fluid. If untreated, will result in ischaemia and the development of proliferative retinopathy.

4   B   **Diagnosis: Retinal detachment**

Painless loss of vision preceded by photopsia with loss of visual field is highly suggestive of retinal detachment. It is more common after trauma and in myopic individuals. Patients often report a dark curtain moving across their vision.

5   D   **Diagnosis: Age-related macular degeneration (ARMD)**

ARMD causes reduction in central macular vision while peripheral vision is preserved. Atrophy of the macula causes a gradual reduction in visual acuity. The retina shows macular drusen.

ENDOCRINOLOGY/METABOLIC

EXTENDED MATCHING QUESTIONS

THEME: OSTEOPOROSIS

1	F	Hip protectors
2	D	Corticosteroids
3	A	Biphosphonates
4	G	Hip protectors
5	G	Hip protectors
6	G	Hip protectors
7	E	Family history

It is well recognised that corticosteroids can cause a fall in bone mass and bone density. HRT is still the treatment of choice for preventing osteoporosis in women under 50 who have had a premature menopause. However, once HRT has been stopped for 10 years, bone density and fracture risk are similar with or without this treatment. The Committee for the Safety of Medicines advise that HRT is no longer the treatment of choice for preventing osteoporosis in women over the age of 50. Bisphosphonates are recommended by NICE to treat post-menopausal women with severe osteoporosis.

There are many risk factors for osteoporosis; family history is an irreversible risk factor.

Hip protectors are effective in reducing the impact of falls, and should be considered for anyone with an increased risk of falls likely to result in fractures or significant injury.

THEME: ENDOCRINE DISEASES

8	A	Acromegaly
9	D	Diabetes insipidus
10	C	Cushing's syndrome
11	B	Conn's syndrome
12	E	Simmond's disease

Cushing's disease and syndrome are associated with excess corticosteroids. Conn's syndrome is caused by excess aldosterone. Diabetes insipidus is due to a deficiency of ADH. Acromegaly is caused by excess growth hormone. Simmond's disease is associated with deficiencies of GH, FSH and LH.

THEME: METABOLIC BONE DISEASE

13	E	Paget's disease
14	G	Rickets
15	C	Osteomalacia
16	B	Hypoparathyroidism
17	E	Paget's disease
18	A	Hyperparathyroidism
19	G	Rickets
20	D	Osteoporosis

You need a good knowledge of general medicine for some questions. Osteoporosis is common and its prevention is a major reason for prescribing HRT. Osteomalacia often presents with bone pain and tenderness and is associated with moderately increased alkaline phosphatase, and decreased calcium and phosphate. Rickets is seen in children and can present with leg and chest deformities. Paget's disease is associated with a hugely increased alkaline phosphatase. It presents as bone pain and tenderness, with bone deformity. The sacrum and lumbar spine are the most commonly affected bones. Paget's disease can be complicated by progressive occlusion of skull foramina, causing deafness, and also by high-output cardiac failure. Hyperparathyroidism is associated with increased calcium levels, bone cysts and subperiosteal erosions in the phalanges. In contrast, hypoparathyroidism is associated with decreased calcium levels but increased phosphate levels, with calcification sometimes seen in the basal ganglia.

THEME: ARTHRITIS

21	**A**	Ankylosing spondylitis
22	**G**	Reiter's syndrome
23	**F**	Psoriatic arthritis
24	**K**	Septic arthritis
25	**C**	Gout
26	**J**	Rubella

Features strongly suggestive of inflammatory spinal disease are insidious onset, onset before 40 years of age, early morning stiffness and improvement with exercise. With suitable treatment prognosis is excellent. There is a 50% chance of passing the HLA B27 gene to offspring and a 33% chance of developing the disease if HLA B27 is positive. Reiter's may start after gastrointestinal infection or urogenital infection. The classic triad of arthritis, conjunctivitis and urethritis is often incomplete. It may be associated with the characteristic skin lesion, keratoderma blenorrhagica. In psoriatic arthropathy the joint activity tends to match the plaque activity. Where nail disease is present, small joint involvement is likely. Septic arthritis usually infects a single joint with pain, fever, erythema and swelling. Gonococcal arthritis is common in women and homosexual men and usually occurs within three weeks of infection. Treatment is with benzylpenicillin. Trauma, surgery, drugs, alcohol or starvation may cause gout. Pseudogout is the deposition of calcium pyrophosphate, typically in the knees. Rubella may cause an acute arthritis similar to rubella, with a positive rheumatoid factor. A self-limiting arthralgia may also be seen with rubella vaccination.

MULTIPLE BEST ANSWER QUESTIONS

1 Gout
Answers: A B E

The annual incidence of gout in the UK is about 1 in 3000 population. The reason for the male preponderance is not known. Two groups of people are particularly affected: obese, male, heavy drinkers of alcohol, and elderly patients taking thiazide diuretics.

2 Hyperuricaemia
Answers: A B D

Hyperuricaemia is induced by furosemide (frusemide), thiazides and polycythaemia rubra vera (due to increased purine turnover). Multiple myeloma is associated with hyperuricaemia due to increased purine turnover but also treatment with antimetabolites causes tissue destruction and a further rise of serum uric acid. There is no such association with diabetes or myxoedema.

3 Hypoglycaemia
Answers: B C D

Alcoholics who do not eat may develop fasting hypoglycaemia due to depletion of glycogen stores by starvation and inhibition of hepatic gluconeogenesis. Other causes include hypopituitarism, Addison's disease, Von Gierke's disease, insulinomas, overtreatment with insulin and severe liver disease. Hepatic carcinomas, mesotheliomas or retroperitoneal fibrosarcomas may cause hypoglycaemia due to secretion of a pro-insulin-like peptide.

4 Pregnancies of diabetic women
Answers: B C E

Diabetic women usually have hydramnios and there is an increased incidence of pre-eclampsia. There is a fourfold increase in congenital abnormalities. Babies born to diabetic women are usually large since insulin has a growth-hormone-like effect in the fetus. The exact cause of increased intra-uterine deaths is unknown.

SINGLE BEST ANSWER QUESTIONS

1 Diabetes Mellitus   **Answers: A**

The diagnosis of diabetes mellitus in a patient with polyuria, thirst and weight loss is confirmed by a random glucose greater or equal to 11.1 mmol/l, a fasting glucose greater or equal to 7.0 mmol/l, or a glucose greater or equal to 11.1 mmol/l two hours after 75 g of glucose in an oral glucose tolerance test.

2 Diabetes Mellitus   **Answers: F**

Standards of the NSF for diabetes include:

- identification of people with diabetes
- empowering people with diabetes
- clinical care of children with diabetes
- clinical care of adults with diabetes
- management of diabetic emergencies
- Prevention of type 2 diabetes is also a standard.

3 Hypothyroidism   **Answer: B**

In a thyroid gland that is failing, the serum T_3 level may remain in the normal range although the serum T_4 level is reduced and serum TSH level elevated. Eventually the serum T_3 level may also fall into the subnormal range. Infiltration of subcutaneous tissues with mucopolysaccharides causes typical facial puffiness, ankle swelling and carpal tunnel syndrome, the last by compression of the median nerve within the flexor retinaculum of the wrist. Pre-tibial myxoedema is a feature of Graves' disease. The macrocytosis occurs in isolation but there is a high incidence of pernicious anaemia in patients with primary hypothyroidism. However, menorrhagia or defective absorption of iron (resulting from achlorhydria) may lead to a microcytic hypochromic anaemia.

4   Carpal tunnel syndrome   Answer: C

In carpal tunnel syndrome, the median nerve may be compressed by changes in the wrist joint (rheumatoid arthritis, acromegaly), soft tissue swelling (myxoedema) or fluid retention (pregnancy). Symptoms are usually worse after a night's rest and improve as activity mobilises extracellular fluid.

SUMMARY COMPLETION QUESTION

THEME: TYPE 2 DIABETES MANAGEMENT

1	H	(prospective)
2	G	(controls)
3	D	(surrogate)
4	A	(reduction)
5	J	($<$)
6	N	(HbA1c)
7	E	(powerful)
8	B	(confounding)

SUMMARY COMPLETION QUESTION

THEME: DIABETES AND COGNITIVE DECLINE

1	G	(association)
2	D	(outcomes)
3	I	(power)
4	B	(narrow)
5	A	(reduce)
6	N	(consistency)
7	K	(undiagnosed)
8	C	(reduces)

PHOTO QUESTION

THEME: HANDS

1   D   Diagnosis: Ganglion

A cystic swelling on the dorsum of the wrist.

2   A   Diagnosis: Swan neck deformity

Hyperextension of the PIP joint with fixed flexion at the DIP joint. This is caused by tendon damage and is typically found in rheumatoid arthritis. Surgical correction may improve functional use.

3   E   Diagnosis: Rheumatoid nodule

Symmetrical synovial swelling is typical of rheumatoid arthritis, typically affecting small joints of the hands or wrists. Often stiff on waking, they improve through the day.

4   B   Diagnosis: Z deformity

This describes hyperextension of the interphalangeal joint with fixed flexion of the metacarpophalangeal joint. It is often seen in rheumatoid arthritis.

5   C   Diagnosis: Heberdens node

Primary nodal osteoarthritis is a common condition particularly affecting elderly women. It causes characteristic nodes on the bases of the distal phalanges.

GASTROENTEROLOGY/NUTRITION

EXTENDED MATCHING QUESTIONS

THEME: CAUSES OF ABDOMINAL PAIN

1	**G**	Pancreatitis
2	**D**	Diverticular disease
3	**E**	Irritable bowel syndrome
4	**F**	Ischaemic colitis
5	**E**	Irritable bowel syndrome
6	**B**	Cholecystitis
7	**C**	Crohn's disease

With clinical scenarios, read the scenario and think about the likely diagnosis in ordinary clinical practice. There will be pointers towards the correct option. Read these scenarios again with the 'correct' answers in mind. In these scenarios, consider the angina and bloody diarrhoea in a 69-year-old as significant and the diagnosis of ischaemic colitis becomes obvious. Similarly, the anal tags and generalised abdominal tenderness point towards Crohn's disease.

THEME: CHANGE IN BOWEL HABIT

8	**I**	Toddler diarrhoea
9	**G**	Irritable bowel syndrome
10	**J**	Ulcerative colitis
11	**A**	Carcinoid syndrome
12	**F**	Hyperthyroidism
13	**B**	Coeliac disease
14	**E**	Giardiasis

Irritable bowel is sometimes considered a diagnosis of exclusion, but diagnostic criteria (Rome and Manning) exist. Patients with ulcerative colitis usually experience symptoms for the first time in their 20s. Long-term surveillance is necessary due to late malignant change. Carcinoid also often produces sharp right hypochondrial pain due to hepatomegaly. Classically, coeliac disease presents as failure to thrive in children. Recently, evidence of coeliac disease has been found in patients presenting to their GPs with vague non-specific symptoms of lethargy and malaise. *Giardia* may be seen not only in travellers but also in gay men, in whom it is sexually transmitted. In some patients it may cause malabsorption.

THEME: INDIGESTION

15 A Alginates

16 H Proton pump inhibitor (PPI)

17 F Misoprostol

18 G Nissen's fundoplication

19 E H_2-receptor antagonist (H_2-RA)

Reflux is common in pregnancy due to progesterone-mediated relaxation of the lower oesophageal sphincter. Alginates such as Gaviscon® are usually sufficient. In the treatment of reflux, mild symptoms should be treated with H_2-RAs or alginates; those proved to have erosive oesophagitis should be treated with PPIs at an initial healing dose and then at a lower dose until a maintenance level is reached. *Helicobacter pylori* treatment is indicated for dyspepsia, not reflux.

MULTIPLE BEST ANSWER QUESTIONS

1 Gallstones   **Answers: B E**

The incidence of stones in the gall bladder rises with age. Many stones remain asymptomatic. Pigment, rather than cholesterol, stones are associated with bacteria in the bile. Chenodeoxycholic acid is ineffective treatment for pigment stones. Cholecystectomy remains the standard treatment for symptomatic gallstones.

2 *Helicobacter pylori*   **Answers: A B**

Helicobacter pylori infection is usually acquired in the first five years of life. The infection is found in about 50% of people over 50, but the rate of infection is decreasing with improved socioeconomic conditions. Infection is associated with duodenal and gastric ulcers, and also gastric carcinoma. Blood tests for *H. pylori* can be confusing because antibodies persist, but the breath test becomes negative once *H. pylori* is eradicated.

3 Acute gastroenteritis   **Answers: A B**

Gastroenteritis in at-risk groups, such as infants and elderly patients, produces dehydration. Oral rehydration therapy (ORT) corrects the dehydration. Commercial preparations are adequate for the treatment of the mild or moderate dehydration commonly seen in the UK. Food has little or no effect on the diarrhoea and should be encouraged as soon as practicable. Antibiotics are rarely required but erythromycin may be needed for *Campylobacter* infection with systemic upset.

4 Crohn's disease   **Answers: A B**

Crohn's disease is a chronic inflammatory disease affecting any part of the gut from the mouth to the anus. It is a transmural inflammation with 'skip lesions' (normal bowel segments). Complications include strictures, fistulae and malabsorption. Anaemia is caused by malabsorption and loss of blood or protein into the bowel. Thrombophlebitis is usually noted with ulcerative colitis.

5 Peptic ulceration   Answers: A E

The association with *H. pylori* infection has been proved and endoscopy is a useful, but not an essential, investigation. Taking milk or food normally relieves pain associated with duodenal ulcer, and vomiting is present only with obstruction. Although proton pump inhibitors are now widely used, H_2 antagonists still have a place.

6 Duodenal ulceration   Answers: A B

There is no evidence to prove a causal relationship between non-steroidal anti-inflammatory drugs and duodenal ulceration. Duodenal ulceration is often a chronic disease with frequent relapses. Duodenal ulceration causes epigastric pain some hours after a meal, when the patient is hungry.

7 Cancer of the colon   Answers: B C D

Early diagnosis is important in cancer of the colon. At present the overall 5-year survival is only 35%. Patients at particular risk of developing cancer of the colon include those with inflammatory bowel disease and patients with a family history of polyposis coli. Patients with a family history of either colonic cancer diagnosed before the age of 45 years or with two first-degree relatives with cancer of the colon are also at increased risk. Screening for faecal occult blood depends on a tumour bleeding, which may occur late in the disease. The test has low sensitivity and specificity.

8 Diverticular disease of the colon   Answers: A B D

A high-fibre diet prevents diverticular disease of the colon. The majority of patients are asymptomatic and do not present to General Practitioners; when symptomatic a high-fibre diet is usually prescribed. Acute diverticulitis is a rare complication, occurring in approximately 1% of affected individuals.

9 Colorectal cancer   Answers: D E

Change in bowel habit can be a feature, but does not need urgent referral, and bleeding with anal symptoms and lower abdominal pain are possible symptoms, but again not requiring urgent referral.
Hb < 11 g/dl in men and an abdominal mass do require urgent referral.

SINGLE BEST ANSWER QUESTIONS

1 Jaundice   **Answer: C**

Jaundice from liver damage is caused by paracetamol, halothane and isoniazid. Arsenic causes fibrosis. Methyldopa interferes with the normal bilirubin pathway. Cholestasis occurs with chlorpromazine and the oral contraceptive pill. The latter can also cause hepatic vein occlusion.

2 Examination of biliary system   **Answer: A**

Oral cholecystography and biliary ultrasound are similar in terms of specificity and sensitivity. The cause of bile duct obstruction can be demonstrated in the majority of cases. However, in about 5% of obstructive jaundice cases the bile ducts are not dilated at the time of examination, especially if the jaundice is not severe or is of short duration. Space-occupying lesions of the liver of about 2 cm in diameter and occasionally 1 cm can be visualised. Metastases, primary liver cancer, cysts or abscesses can be identified. Ultrasonography also demonstrates ascites.

3 Irritable bowel syndrome   **Answer: A**

A significant minority of patients relate their symptoms, usually of painless diarrhoea, to an episode of infective diarrhoea, often contracted abroad. The whole gut may be involved and gastric symptoms may coexist with colonic ones. A barium enema on colonoscopy is not essential in most patients, especially when all the typical features are present in the young person. The diagnosis is common in the elderly but more extensive investigations are required to rule out alternative diagnoses. Despite the similarities between the irritable bowel syndrome and diverticular disease, evidence is lacking that irritable bowel syndrome precedes diverticular disease in individuals.

4 Drugs causing constipation   **Answer: D**

Aluminium trisilicate, tricyclic antidepressants and oral contraceptives may cause constipation. Iron most commonly causes constipation but it can also cause diarrhoea. Cimetidine causes diarrhoea rather than constipation.

5   Irritable bowel syndrome   **Answer: A**

Irritable bowel syndrome (IBS) most commonly presents in the mid 30s,
patients are seldom over 50 years. Symptoms of IBS are common in
childhood and many adults with IBS give a history which extends back
to childhood.

6   Diverticular disease   **Answer: D**

Diverticular disease is the clinical syndrome which complicates
diverticulosis, so by definition it cannot occur without symptoms. The
sigmoid colon is the most common segment of the bowel to be affected
by diverticular disease. Rectal bleeding seldom occurs, but when it
does it usually settles spontaneously without treatment. The treatment
for acute diverticular disease is hospitalisation, rest, analgesia (avoiding
morphine) and antibiotics, including metronidazole. Surgery is rarely
necessary acutely.

PHOTO QUESTION

THEME: MISCELLANEOUS

1   B   Diagnosis: Parotid cyst

A short history of parotid swelling requires urgent assessment and cytology to exclude malignancy.

2   E   Diagnosis: ITP

This photo shows thrombocytopenic purpura on the tongue and buccal mucosa. Urgent confirmation of platelet count and haematological referral are needed to avoid haemorrhage.

3   A   Diagnosis: Entropion

This photo shows a lower lid entropion with irritation of the conjunctiva. This may result in bacterial conjunctivitis and an unpleasant foreign body sensation.

4   D   Diagnosis: Geographical tongue

This benign condition is of no clinical significance and requires no more than reassurance.

5   C   Diagnosis: Naevus

Naevi that are suspicious should be excised and sent for histological examination to confirm both diagnosis and complete excision.

INFECTIOUS DISEASES/ HAEMATOLOGY/IMMUNOLOGY/ ALLERGIES/GENETICS

EXTENDED MATCHING QUESTIONS

THEME: TREATMENT OF INFLUENZA

1	**D**	Neuraminidase inhibitors
2	**D**	Neuraminidase inhibitors
3	**G**	Vaccination
4	**G**	Vaccination
5	**H**	Zanamivir
6	**H**	Zanamivir

Vaccination the most important measure for reducing mortality and morbidity in high-risk groups.

Neuraminidase inhibitors as a group have been shown to be clinically effective for the treatment of influenza in otherwise healthy adults and, when taken as prophylaxis, decrease the likelihood of developing influenza by over 70%. Zanamivir is now recommended by NICE for the treatment of at-risk adults when influenza is in the community and the patient has presented within 36 hours of developing symptoms. Zanamivir has to be taken as an inhaler or nasal spray, whereas oseltamivir can be given orally.

THEME: CHROMOSOME DISORDERS

7 C X-linked

8 A Autosomal dominant

9 B Autosomal recessive

10 C X-linked

11 A Autosomal dominant

Haemophilia (A and B) is a sex-linked disease, as is red–green colour blindness. These problems will therefore only rarely (but not never) be seen in females. Familial hypercholesterolaemia is one of the commonest inherited disorders in the West, and is autosomal dominant. Familial adenomatous polyposis coli is uncommon, accounting for about 1% of all colon cancers. It is inherited as an autosomal dominant disorder. Cystic fibrosis is one of the commonest autosomal recessive conditions.

THEME: INFECTIVE AGENTS ASSOCIATED WITH TUMOURS

12 B *Helicobacter pylori*

13 C Hepatitis B virus

14 D Human herpesvirus type 8

15 E Human papillomavirus

16 E Human papillomavirus

Primary gastric lymphoma is strongly associated with *Helicobacter pylori* infection. The development of hepatocellular carcinoma is linked with the hepatitis B virus. Kaposi's sarcoma is common in patients with AIDS and there is a firm association with human herpesvirus type 8. All warts are benign tumours and caused by human papillomavirus (HPV). Genital warts are caused by HPV types 6 and 11. Other HPV serotypes, especially 16 and 18, have been implicated in the development of cervical intraepithelial neoplasia and invasive cervical cancer.

MULTIPLE BEST ANSWER QUESTIONS

1   Turner's syndrome   **Answers: A B**

Turner's syndrome (XO genotype) is frequently associated with coarctation of the aorta, streak gonads, primary amenorrhoea and short stature. It is commonly seen in spontaneous abortions. They have neck webbing and an increased carrying angle at the elbow.

2   Pertussis immunisation   **Answers: B D**

Absolute contraindications to pertussis immunisation are:

- Severe general reactions: fever equal to or more than 39.5 °C within 48 hours of vaccine; anaphylaxis; generalised collapse; prolonged unresponsiveness; prolonged inconsolable screaming; and convulsions occurring within 72 hours

- Severe local reaction to the preceding dose: an area of extensive redness and swelling which becomes indurated and involves most of the antero-lateral area of the thigh or the major part of the circumference of the upper arm

- Unstable neurological condition: unlike symptomatic hypoglycaemic fits, the outcome of hypocalcaemic fits in the neonatal period is usually good and not associated with neurodevelopmental problems

3   Infectious hepatitis   **Answers: B C**

Hepatitis C (previously called non-A, non-B hepatitis) is now the commonest blood-borne hepatitis in the UK. Hepatitis D (delta agent) coexists with hepatitis B and is relatively rare in the UK. Hepatitis E is food/water-borne, producing an illness similar to hepatitis A. It is hoped the widespread vaccination against hepatitis B will greatly reduce the incidence of primary hepatoma.

4   Glandular fever   Answers: A B E

In glandular fever, liver function tests are abnormal in over 80% but less than 10% are jaundiced. If given ampicillin, patients will develop a rash. The sore throat lasts for more than seven days. Patients can have prolonged lethargy and depression for many months after the acute illness. About 80% of patients have a positive monospot test. Antibody production may be slow and you may need to repeat the test in two weeks to confirm the diagnosis.

5   Normal iron metabolism   Answers: A C

The normal daily requirement for adults is 1–2 mg. Haemoglobin accounts for about 75% of total body iron. Haem iron, present in meat, is more readily absorbed than inorganic iron. Although inorganic iron usually predominates in the diet, relatively little can be made available for absorption, the exact amount depending on the presence or absence of dietary components and gastrointestinal secretions that enhance the solubility of iron. There is no physiological route for iron excretion.

6   Pneumococcal immunisation   Answers: A C

Pneumococcal immunisation should be considered for all those in whom pneumococcal infection is more common or more serious. This includes patients with homozygous sickle cell disease, asplenia and chronic renal, cardiac, liver or respiratory disease. In HIV-positive patients, the serological response to vaccination, and hence benefit, declines with the increased immunocompromised state. Routine revaccination is not normally recommended.

7   Pneumococcal infections   Answers: B D F

There is a need to consider pneumococcal vaccination in patients with multiple myeloma, sickle cell disease and post-splenectomy.

SINGLE BEST ANSWER QUESTIONS

1 Measles   **Answer: B**

The respiratory complications of measles include pneumonia, bronchiolitis and bronchiectasis but not recurrent pneumothoraces. Corneal ulceration may occur. Severe infection from prolonged and intense exposure to infected siblings in the same household is more likely than malnutrition to cause fatal disease. Lifelong immunity is established after natural infection.

2 Depressed immune response   **Answer: A**

Malnutrition rather than obesity may cause a depressed immune response. Extremes of life represent periods of increased risk from infection. For example, the elderly are particularly susceptible to pneumococcal pneumonia. Certain infections depress the immune response, as in AIDS.

3 Red blood cell macrocytosis   **Answer: B**

The macrocytosis of coeliac disease is usually due to folate deficiency. Alcohol makes the red cells large directly, through secondary folate deficiency and because of liver disease. In aplasia, younger larger red cells leave the bone marrow.

4 Haematological conditions   **Answer: D**

Iron deficiency is linked with microcytic anaemia, as are vitamins A and C and pyridoxine deficiencies. Cobalamin deficiency is linked to megaloblastic anaemia, as is folic acid deficiency.

5 Sickle cell anaemia   **Answer: B**

Folic acid deficiency may increase aplastic crises and folate supplements are recommended, particularly during pregnancy when crisis frequency may increase. There is chronic haemolysis which results in normal or raised serum iron levels. Recurrent tissue infarcts lead to splenic fibrosis and shrinkage, pulmonary hypertension and focal neurological signs. Recurrent haematuria, occasionally nephrotic syndrome, aseptic femoral head necrosis and priapism may all occur. Septic complications are most frequent and life threatening. Pneumococcal septicaemia is a major hazard because of hyposplenism. Prophylactic penicillin and immunisation are used.

6 Complications of rheumatoid disease   Answer: A

Finger clubbing is not associated with rheumatoid disease but swan-neck deformities of the fingers are recognised signs. The systemic manifestations include pericarditis, pleurisy and weight loss. Baker's synovial cysts occur due to joint complications and leg ulcers are due to arteritis. Pernicious anaemia is an associated autoimmune disease.

PHOTO QUESTION

THEME: INFECTION

1   E   Diagnosis: Infection

This patient developed a local infection in one of his skin lesions after an episode of minor trauma. It settled quickly with flucloxacillin.

2   D   Diagnosis: Sebaceous cyst

This photo shows the characteristic appearance of a sebaceous cyst with the keratin plug clearly visible.

3   C   Diagnosis: Ringworm

This photo demonstrates the annular spreading appearance of ringworm.

4   B   Diagnosis: Shingles

The unmistakeable vesicular appearance on a background of erythema with pain is pathognomonic of shingles. Prompt treatment with oral antivirals may be effective in shortening the duration of symptoms.

5   A   Diagnosis: Haematuria

In the presence of symptoms of dysuria and frequency, haematuria is often the result of infection, and in most areas trimethoprim is a first-line treatment of choice. In painless haematuria investigation of the renal tract is indicated.

PAEDIATRICS

EXTENDED MATCHING QUESTIONS

THEME: COMMON DEVELOPMENTAL MILESTONES

1   D   12 months

2   C   9 months

3   E   18 months

4   E   18 months

5   B   6 months

6   A   3 months

7   D   12 months

You will need a good grasp of children's developmental milestones. At 3 months, babies can be pulled to sitting with little head lag and will hold an object placed in the hand. At 6 months, babies sit supported and transfer a cube between hands. At 9 months, they sit unsupported and may crawl on the abdomen. At 12 months, they walk with one hand held and say two to three words with meaning. At 18 months, they will manage a spoon, build a three- to four-cube tower, and say 10–12 words with meaning.

THEME: ABDOMINAL PAIN IN CHILDREN

8   G   Henoch-Schönlein purpura (HSP)

9   D   Intussusception

10   H   Appendicitis

11   J   Testicular torsion

12   L   Mesenteric adenitis

The purpura in HSP is classically found on extensor surfaces of the lower limbs. Treatment is supportive. The classic presentation of intussusception is rare, and it may present initially like gastroenteritis. If the appendix is retrocaecal or pelvic, appendicitis may present as diarrhoea or dysuria. Urine should always be tested in children with abdominal pain. All boys with abdominal pain must have their testes examined. The danger of small bowel strangulation with inguinal hernia is high and these cases should always be referred urgently. Diabetic ketoacidosis may cause abdominal pain which resolves on treatment with fluids and insulin.

MULTIPLE BEST ANSWER QUESTIONS

1   Sudden infant death syndrome   **Answers: C E F**

Important risk factors for sudden infant death syndrome include male sex, prone sleeping position, the winter months and respiratory symptoms. Maternal factors include high parity, young maternal age and smoking.

2   Breast-feeding   **Answers: A B C**

Breast-feeding protects against respiratory disease and gastrointestinal infections. It reduces the risk of insulin-dependent diabetes and maternal breast cancer. Childhood obesity is less likely to be found in breast-fed infants.

3   Breast-fed babies   **Answers: A C E**

Breast-fed babies are less likely to have gastroenteritis but there is no known association with coeliac disease. Urinary tract infections are usually associated with vesicoureteric reflux. There is a decreased incidence of non-accidental injury, cot death and eczema in breast-fed babies, who are also less likely to be obese.

4   Down's syndrome   **Answers: A C D**

Features in 75% of people with Down's syndrome include upslanting palpebral fissures, flat facies, flat occiput and loose skin on the neck. Features in 50% of people with Down's syndrome include broad hands, short fingers, incurved fifth finger (clinodactyly), single palmar crease, malformed auricles, Brushfield's spots, protruding tongue, hypotonia and broad space between first and second toes. The IQ is usually between 20 and 70, average 50.

5   Congenital dislocation of the hip   Answers: C D E

Congenital dislocation of the hip is four times more common in girls than in boys. In doing Ortolani's test it is essential to abduct to 90°: less than 70° abduction is abnormal. It is sometimes picked up because of delayed walking and treatment at this stage normally requires open reduction. The best time to pick up dislocation is as soon after birth as possible, as treatment using a frog plaster is always effective.

6   Down's syndrome   Answers: B D

People with Down's syndrome are prone to hypothyroidism. Clinical recognition is difficult because people with Down's syndrome are shorter than average, slower, less active and less alert and occasionally have a hoarse voice. Post-mortem studies of people with Down's syndrome have confirmed that a high proportion have pathological changes indistinguishable from Alzheimer's disease.

7   Nocturnal enuresis   Answers: A C

Ninety per cent of children with nocturnal enuresis are dry during the day. First-born children appear to be more prone to nocturnal enuresis than later children. By the age of 10 years, 7% of children still wet their beds at least once a week. Urodynamic studies do not often help diagnose the cause of nocturnal enuresis. It is not known how the tricyclic antidepressants (eg imipramine) achieve temporary dryness, but it does not seem to be related to their anticholinergic or antidepressant effect or their local anaesthetic effects on the bladder.

8   Baby of 8 months   Answers: A C

Rolling over is acquired by most babies at 5 months of age. The ability to pick up a bead between finger and thumb is usually only evident at about 1 year. Babies sit unsupported at 8 months. Babies usually feed themselves with a spoon after 1 year. Most babies say their first words clearly around 12–14 months, but five words will often not be clearly spoken until 14–16 months.

SINGLE BEST ANSWER QUESTIONS

1 Congenital dislocation of the hip   **Answer: C**

The incidence of congenital dislocation of the hip is 2–3 per 1000 births. Screening may not be worthwhile – the rate of surgical intervention has not decreased with screening. Splinting can be associated with avascular necrosis of the femoral head.

2 Congenital dislocation of the hip   **Answer: A**

Congenital dislocation of hips is seen in about 0.25% of newborns with a female-to-male predominance of 8:1. Most are unilateral and usually are on the left. Ninety per cent of dislocatable hips will stabilise in the first two months of life. However, the ones which will stabilise cannot be predicted, so all patients are treated with a flexion-abduction-external rotation device. Ultrasound of the hips is very useful in making the diagnosis in the newborn. Femoral head ossification centres appear at three to six months so radiographs are not useful in the newborn. The most significant risk factor for hip dysplasia is a positive family history. Other risk factors for hip dysplasia include breech presentation, foot deformities, oligohydramnios, primiparity and female sex.

3 Puberty   **Answer: A**

Menarche is a late event in puberty. On average, there is only 2 inches (5 cm) of growth potential remaining after the menarche. The pubertal growth spurt in normal girls always occurs earlier. Delayed pubertal development is most commonly due to physiological delay in development, hallmarked by short stature, delayed adrenarche, delayed gonadarche and a retarded bone age. The commonest cause of central precocious puberty in girls is 'idiopathic'. In boys the commonest cause is a CNS lesion.

PHOTO QUESTION

THEME: LOWER LIMBS

1   D   Diagnosis: Pyoderma

This is an uncommon condition occasionally seen in diabetics, which often starts as a sterile ulcer. This patient had these lesions for many years and the initial ulceration has been replaced by scar tissue.

2   B   Diagnosis: Varicose veins

These impressive varicose veins will inevitably result in chronic venous hypertension unless they are controlled surgically or through the use of support hosiery.

3   A   Diagnosis: Café au lait patches

These are one feature of neurofibromatosis. Other features include soft tissue neurofibromas and occasionally acoustic neuromas, phaeochromocytomas and schwannomas.

4   C   Diagnosis: Osteoarthritis

This unfortunate gentleman broke his legs in a collision between the tank he was a passenger in and a German artillery shell. Surgery restored his mobility but the resulting anatomical asymmetry has resulted in progressive genu valgum and secondary arthritis.

5   E   Diagnosis: Ischaemic toe

The finding of isolated embolic disease should prompt a search for the source of the emboli. Common culprits include the major arteries of the legs, the aorta and the heart, particularly atrial fibrillation.

PHARMACO-THERAPEUTICS

EXTENDED MATCHING QUESTIONS

THEME: COMPLEMENTARY MEDICINE

1	H	Saw palmetto
2	A	Angus castus
3	G	St John's wort
4	F	Ginkgo
5	G	St John's wort
6	B	Butterbur

All practitioners should have some knowledge about complementary medicine. Saw palmetto appears to be effective in the treatment of benign prostatic hypertrophy, and angus castus seems to be effective in relieving symptoms of pre-menstrual syndrome.

St John's wort is very popular. It is used in depression. However St John's wort has numerous drug interactions, and because it is a liver enzyme inducer it can reduce the level of the oral contraceptive pill.

Ginkgo has been used in memory loss and dementia, but should be avoided in people taking aspirin and warfarin since it inhibits a platelet-activating factor.

Butterbur is often useful in the treatment of hayfever.

THEME: SIMILAR-SOUNDING DRUGS

7	E	Loratadine
8	C	Loperamide
9	A	Lansoprazole
10	D	Loprazolam
11	F	Lorazepam

12 E   Loratadine

13 A   Lansoprazole

14 B   Lofepramine

Some questions about drugs can be answered easily. Loratadine is an antihistamine and can be used in the symptomatic treatment of urticaria. Loperamide is used as an adjunct to rehydration in acute diarrhoea and can cause abdominal cramps. Lansoprazole is a proton pump inhibitor and can be used in the treatment of duodenal ulcers. Loprazolam is a hypnotic. Lorazepam is an anxiolytic and can be used in the treatment of status epilepticus. Lofepramine is an antidepressant.

THEME: SIDE-EFFECTS OF DYSPEPSIA TREATMENT

15 E   Misoprostol

16 E   Misoprostol

17 C   Magnesium salts

18 F   Omeprazole

19 A   Aluminium salts

20 D   Metoclopramide

21 D   Metoclopramide

22 B H_2-receptor antagonists

The side-effects of common treatments ought to be familiar. Misoprostol can cause inter-menstrual bleeding and can be associated with post-menopausal bleeding. Aluminium salts frequently cause constipation, while magnesium salts are frequently associated with diarrhoea. Omeprazole can cause severe skin reactions and photosensitivity. Metoclopramide is associated with dystonic reactions and can cause galactorrhoea. H_2-receptor antagonists can cause confusion, which is reversible on stopping the medication.

THEME: ANTI-INFECTIVE DRUG SIDE-EFFECTS

23 A   Aciclovir

24 H   Zanamavir

25 D   Doxycycline

26 F   Rifampicin

27 C   Ciprofloxacin

28 E   Metronidazole

Long-term treatment with aciclovir in the prophylaxis of recurrent herpes simplex infections requires regular monitoring of renal function. Zanamavir (Relenza®) should not be used in severe asthmatics and patients with mild asthma should be advised to keep a bronchodilator to hand. Patients on doxycycline should be warned about the risk of sunburn, particularly when used for malarial prophylaxis. Patients being treated for TB or given meningococcal prophylaxis should be warned about staining of contact lenses. The elderly and those on steroids are particularly prone to tendon damage. The Committee on the Safety of Medicines (CSM) advise stopping quinolones at the first signs of tendon inflammation. They are contraindicated in pregnant women and children. Metronidazole may cause severe nausea and vomiting if taken with alcohol. Ciprofloxacin may potentiate the effects of alcohol.

MULTIPLE BEST ANSWER QUESTIONS

1 Renal failure   Answers: B E

Tetracyclines, apart from doxycycline, should be avoided in renal failure as they are anti-anabolic, causing salt and water loss, raise the blood urea and can lead to permanent loss of nephrons in the kidney. Nitrofurantoin is prone to reach toxic levels and cause peripheral neuropathy in renal failure. It is also likely to be ineffective for urinary infections. Although aluminium hydroxide is used for phosphate lowering, there are concerns about aluminium retention with prolonged usage.

2 Benzodiazepine anxiolytics   Answers: B D

There is little difference in the pharmacodynamics of the many available benzodiazepines. They do, however, differ in their duration of action. Temazepam and oxazepam are short-acting, whereas diazepam and its active metabolites persist in the body for a long time with a half-life of up to three days in the elderly. The increase in body sway predisposes to falls, especially in the elderly.

3 Cannabis   Answers: A D

Cannabis is usually smoked but can be ingested or injected intravenously. The clinical features of cannabis intake include euphoria with drowsiness, distorted and heightened images, altered tactile sensations, tachycardia, hypertension and ataxia with visual and auditory hallucinations. Injections may produce nausea and vomiting within minutes and, after about an hour, profuse watery diarrhoea.

4 Aspirin   Answers: A C

Aspirin in large doses is hypoprothrombinaemic. In smaller doses, it increases the bleeding tendency by its antiplatelet and gastric irritant effects. Also, in large doses, aspirin is uricosuric, but in therapeutic doses of 1–2 g/day or less, it reduces urate excretion.

5 Renal failure   Answers: A C E

Aspirin causes sodium and water retention, deterioration in renal function and increased risk of gastrointestinal bleeding. Avoid glibenclamide in severe renal impairment, because of increased risk of hypoglycaemia. Muscle toxicities may occur with all statins, particularly in patients with renal impairment.

6 Cannabis abuse   Answers: C D

Chronic cannabis abuse produces reversible intellectual impairment. Initial reports of cerebral atrophy have not been confirmed. Cannabis smoke may be carcinogenic.

7 Side-effects of benzodiazepines   Answers: A B C

Benzodiazepines are anxiolytic, sedative anticonvulsants and act as muscle relaxants. Benzodiazepines are well tolerated and side-effects tend to be a result of overdosage, which leads to drowsiness and confused thinking, especially in the elderly. They potentiate the effects of central nervous system depressants such as alcohol.

8 Warfarin   Answers: A D E

The main interactions with warfarin are due either to hepatic enzyme inhibition (eg cimetidine, co-trimoxazole) or to enzyme induction (eg rifampicin, phenytoin). Non-steroidal anti-inflammatory drugs may predispose to gastric erosion and ulceration, with consequent risk of gastrointestinal bleeding.

9 Combined oral contraceptive pill   Answers: A B E

The effectiveness of the combined pill can be reduced by antibiotics, some tranquillisers and anticonvulsants, and griseofulvin. Rifamycin accelerates metabolism of the Pill and reduces its effect, as do carbamazepine and griseofulvin. The Pill antagonises the anticoagulant effect of warfarin and antagonises the hypotensive effect of lisinopril.

10   Non-steroidal anti-inflammatory drugs   **Answers: D E**

Hyperkalaemia is linked with non-steroidal anti-inflammatory drugs (NSAIDs). Haemolytic anaemia, rather than polycythaemia, is linked with usage of NSAIDs.

SINGLE BEST ANSWER QUESTIONS

1   Drugs contraindicated in breast-feeding   **Answer: B**

Most drugs enter breast milk by passive lipid diffusion. As the plasma drug concentration is relatively low compared to total body concentration, the load to the baby is small. It is wise to be cautious, but only drugs known to be toxic to the child should be avoided completely. Senna can cause increased gastric mobility and diarrhoea.

2   Zanamivir (Relenza®)   **Answer: B**

Zanamivir probably affects neuraminidase activity and so inhibits replication of influenza virus (types A and B). It has to be taken as a nasal spray or dry powder inhalation, and its effect is greatest in those patients seen within 30 hours. It does enable a quicker return to work but may possibly exacerbate asthma.

3   St. John's wort   **Answer: A**

St John's wort is used commonly in the UK, and has been shown to be effective in treating depression. It can induce liver enzymes and can interact with digoxin, warfarin and the Pill.

4   Digoxin therapy   **Answer: D**

Old people are at risk of toxicity, especially with hypokalaemia or hypercalcaemia. Almost any arrhythmia (usually SVT with AV block) will occur. Other symptoms include decreased cognition, yellow-green visual halos, nausea and vomiting. Prolonged PR interval is noted with first-degree heart block.

5 Warfarin   **Answer: D**

All broad-spectrum antibiotics, including ampicillin, can increase the prothrombin time. In drug interactions with warfarin, consider these effects:

- Displacement of warfarin from the protein-binding site by, for example, sulphonamides, NSAIDs and sulphonylureas. A new steady state is then established. Consequently, the danger is at the start or end of therapy.
- Enzyme inhibition or competition (eg cimetidine).
- Enzyme induction (eg rifampicin, griseofulvin and carbamazepine).

6 Glibenclamide   **Answer: A**

Glibenclamide has a relatively long biological half-life although it is shorter than chlorpropamide. Unfortunately, it also has biologically active metabolites with a long half-life that are excreted by the kidney. This therefore precludes the use of glibenclamide in patients with renal impairment. It should be used with caution in the elderly. Despite strong protein binding, all sulphonylureas cross the placenta, producing fetal hyperinsulinaemia and predisposing to acrosomia and neonatal hypoglycaemia.

PSYCHIATRY/NEUROLOGY

EXTENDED MATCHING QUESTIONS

THEME: SECTIONS OF THE MENTAL HEALTH ACT

1 **E** Section 7

2 **B** Section 3

3 **C** Section 4

4 **D** Section 5

5 **A** Section 2

Some knowledge of the Mental Health Act is desirable. Section 2 is used for assessment, section 3 for treatment. Sections 4 and 5 are both emergency detention orders; Section 4 is used to admit someone to hospital; and Section 5 is used to keep someone in hospital. Section 7 is concerned with guardianship.

THEME: HEADACHES

6 **B** Migraine

7 **D** Tension headache

8 **D** Tension headache

9 **B** Migraine

10 **A** Cluster headache

Patients with tension headache often describe the pain as a 'weight on the top of the head' or as a 'band'. Headache that is pain referred from the neck may be associated with certain movements, postures or positions. With migraine the patient will commonly show pallor and often experiences flushing. Cluster headaches are frequently accompanied by the complaint of a watery eye.

THEME: DISC LESIONS

11 B   At L5–S1 level

12 C   Central disc prolapse

13 A   At L2–L3 level

Patients with disc lesions at the L2–L3 level will usually demonstrate a positive femoral stretch test. At the L5–S1 level there will be loss of the ankle reflex. With a central disc prolapse there will usually be loss of bladder function.

THEME: QUESTIONNAIRES

14 A   CAGE

15 E   SCOFF

16 D   MAST

17 A   CAGE

MAST and CAGE are commonly used questionnaires in detecting alcohol problems. MAST asks 10 questions and has a maximum score of 32. The questions include ones about alcohol-related driving and hospital admissions. CAGE is a very short questionnaire with only four questions, but it is significant if any two questions are positive. SCOFF is used in eating disorders. EAT is not a questionnaire: it is an Employment Appeal Tribunal.

THEME: HEADACHE

18 G¹   Tension headache

19 C   Coital cephalgia

20 B   Cluster headache

21 E   Migraine without aura

22 F H   Temporal arteritis

23 D   Migraine with aura

One of the key points in the history of tension headache is that it occurs at times of stress and gets better on relaxation, eg on holiday. Coital cephalgia is rare and onset is during intercourse. The clinical picture may be similar to that of subarachnoid haemorrhage and CSF examination may be necessary to differentiate between the two. Cluster headache is seen in a sex ratio of 7:1, male:female, and produces bouts of pain 20–60 minutes long, occurring at the same time each day. There may be associated facial flushing, nasal secretion or even an ipsilateral Horner's syndrome. Alcohol may provoke attacks. Giant cell arteritis typically affects the elderly who may present with symptoms of polymyalgia rheumatica. Early diagnosis and treatment with high-dose steroids is crucial in preserving sight.

THEME: PSYCHIATRIC COMPLAINTS

24 E   Dementia

25 D   Conversion disorder

26 A   Anxiety disorder

27 C   Borderline personality disorder

28 B   Bipolar disorder

29 J   Schizophrenia

Dementia typically causes loss of short-term memory first, and socially skilled patients may confabulate to get around this. Mood disorders may appear and family relationships are often strained by their inability to carry out simple tasks. Conversion disorder often represents a patient's idea of what the disease looks like, hence symptoms and signs seldom match. There is usually some gain for the patient and they may seem remarkably unfazed by events, 'la belle indifference'. Anxiety disorders often start after a stressful life event, and attacks consist of psychological symptoms of fearful anticipation and worry, and physical symptoms. The symptoms of borderline personality disorder are similar to those of antisocial personality disorder. The symptoms of the manic phase in bipolar disorder are similar in some respects to hyperthyroidism and this should be excluded.

THEME: MIGRAINE

30 **A** Aspirin

31 **B** Avoidance of trigger factors

32 **G** PR diclofenac

33 **I** Sumatriptan

34 **E** Ergotamine

35 **D** Emergency medical referral

A stepwise approach to migraine treatment starts with over-the-counter remedies such as aspirin as step 1. Step 2 involves parenteral routes. If migraines are not controlled on this step the next treatment is sumatriptan. If sumatriptan does not control symptoms the diagnosis should be reviewed. Ergotamine is a step-4 treatment. At any time alternative diagnoses should be considered, particularly subarachnoid haemorrhage or meningitis. Opiates and opioids should never be used due to potential for addiction and poor efficacy.

THEME: HEADACHES

36 **G** Temporal arteritis

37 **F** Migraine

38 **A** Alcoholism

39 **E** Depression

40 **C** Carbon monoxide poisoning

The answer requires the most likely diagnosis. Each of the histories could possibly have more than one answer, but the question is specific. Although the middle-aged GP may have a brain tumour, it is far more likely that he is a drinker. The young girl moving in with her boyfriend is possibly going to get migraine from and the oral contraceptive pill, and the patient who has just moved house may have a faulty central heating boiler.

THEME: MRC SCALE FOR MUSCLE POWER

41 **E**   3

42 **C**   1

43 **H**   5

In the MRC scale for muscle power, 5 = normal power, 3 = movement overcomes gravity plus added resistance, and 1 = no movement of joint but muscle contraction visible.

THEME: NERVE ROOT LESIONS

44 **G**   S1/S2

45 **B**   C5

46 **C**   C6

47 **E**   L3/4

You need to know about innervations of reflexes and muscles. Although these can vary somewhat the clinical scenarios will be specific.

Biceps reflex = C5

Supinator reflex = C6

Triceps reflex = C6/C7

Knee reflex = L3/L4

Ankle reflex = S1

MULTIPLE BEST ANSWER QUESTIONS

1   Bulimia nervosa   **Answers: A E**

Bulimia nervosa is characterised by frequent binges, behaviour such as vomiting or fasting to prevent weight gain, and over concern about shape and weight.

2   Essential tremor   **Answers: B D**

Essential tremor is most pronounced with outstretched arms (sustained posture) and is typically relieved by alcohol. A Parkinson's disease tremor is most pronounced at rest and is a cerebellar tremor with movement (intention). Anxiety may exacerbate both essential and Parkinson's disease tremor.

3   Risk factors for suicide   **Answers: A D E F**

Risk factors for suicide include a history of recent self-harm, the severity of depressive illness, and the presence of active plans. Being male, unemployed and single are also risk factors.

4   Major depression   **Answers: B C E**

A working class background predisposes to major depression. The loss of a parent in childhood and the presence of several children in the house also predispose to an episode of major depression. Unemployment, rather than continuous employment, is a major factor in the aetiology of depression.

5   Compensation neurosis   **Answers: B E**

The incidence of compensation neurosis has an inverse relationship with the severity of the injury. It is twice as common after industrial injuries as after road traffic accidents. Little recovery is found in patients with severe symptoms even after settlement of the compensation claim. The main symptoms are headaches, dizziness, poor concentration and irritability. Malingering is not a common occurrence, and the mechanisms involved in producing these symptoms appear to be subconscious ones.

6   Agoraphobia   **Answers: B C D**

Agoraphobia generally commences suddenly in adult life following a recent traumatic event. There is a large preponderance of women patients, and a worsening of symptoms can occur as a result of other emotional changes such as a period of depression. Treatment is very difficult, but the condition can respond to desensitisation by systematically introducing the patient to the feared situation.

7   Grief reaction   **Answers: A B D**

The initial stage of a grief reaction is a period of numbness with little or no emotional reaction. This is the period of denial. Subsequent stages follow to a state of depression, and suicidal ideas are often expressed. These may reflect feelings of guilt or identification with the dead person. The reaction is self-limiting although there may be delays of up to several years. The treatment of choice would be some form of psychotherapy or counselling. The grief reaction is a neurotic illness rather than psychotic.

8   Anxiety states   **Answers: A E**

Many physical symptoms are associated with anxiety states: dyspnoea, difficulty inhaling, overbreathing, dry mouth, difficulty swallowing, palpitations, chest pain, frequency and urgency of micturition, tinnitus, blurred vision, paraesthesia, dizziness and sweating. Difficulty concentrating and complaints of poor memory occur. Persistent and objective memory loss is not present and raises the possibility of an organic cause. Depressive illnesses may present with anxiety symptoms: low mood and early morning wakening would be indicative of this. Problems getting to sleep are more usual with anxiety disorders.

9   Obsessive-compulsive disorder   Answers: A E

Obsessive-compulsive disorders are characterised by obsessional
thinking and compulsive behaviour. Obsessional thoughts are words,
ideas or beliefs that intrude into the patient's mind. They are recognised
as the patient's own thoughts. They are usually unpleasant, are resisted
and are associated with anxiety. Obsessional thoughts lead to
obsessional actions which may reduce anxiety. Obsessional ruminations
are endless internal debates, sometimes about insignificant details.
Anxiety and depression are commonly associated. Men and women are
equally affected. Two-thirds improve by the end of a year; cases lasting
more than one year run a fluctuating course.

10 Schizophrenia   Answers: A D E

In the absence of coarse brain disease the presence of Schneider's first-
rank symptoms point to a diagnosis of schizophrenia. They are:

- Specific types of auditory hallucination (audible thoughts,
  voices talking about the patient in the third person, voices
  commenting on actions (running commentary))

- Passivity phenomena (breakdown of ego-boundaries), thought
  insertion, withdrawal and broadcast, forced acts and feelings
  (somatic passivity)

- Delusions (primary delusions or delusional perceptions).

11 Acute confusional state   Answers: C D E

Almost every disease, bodily insult and drug has been credited with
precipitating acute confusion. Commonly implicated factors are trauma,
surgery, heart failure, infection, anoxia and sedative drugs. Confusion is
not, however, a characteristic feature of myxoedema. Dementia is a
very common predisposing condition and tricyclics may precipitate a
confusional state. Phenothiazines such as thioridazine may be used
therapeutically but dealing with the precipitating factor is most
important.

12 Hypomania

Answers: A C E

Flight of ideas, where there is an excessively fluent flow of thoughts and ideas, but with some thread of connection between them, is characteristic of hypomania. Thought insertion is a first-rank symptom of schizophrenia. Overactivity and a sense of grandiosity can lead to sexually promiscuous behaviour. Delusions of bodily illness are a feature of depression, not mania. The manic patient is so active he/she tends to have very little sleep and can become ill through exhaustion.

13 Alcohol withdrawal

Answers: A B D

Delirium tremens on withdrawal from alcohol includes a coarse, persistent tremor of the hands. Often, the patient experiences visual hallucinations, such as seeing animals crawling on the floor or the bedclothes. There is free perspiration, oliguria and dehydration. Passivity feelings are features of schizophrenia. Confabulation is part of Korsakoff's syndrome, which results from chronic alcohol abuse and is not a feature of acute withdrawal.

14 Hysteria

Answers: B C

A hysterical symptom is one that suggests physical illness but occurs in the absence of physical disease and is not produced deliberately. Hysterical symptoms occur in association with several psychiatric disorders: depression, anxiety and organic mental disorder. 'La belle indifference' is a characteristic, but is not always present. Hysterical symptoms developing for the first time in middle or old age should raise a high suspicion of organic disease. There are usually obvious discrepancies between signs and symptoms of hysteria and those of organic disease, although this depends on the patient's medical knowledge.

15 Suicide   **Answers: A D F G**

Tactful enquiry about suicidal intent may decrease the risk of suicide. The following factors are associated with an increased risk of suicide: male sex, old age, alcohol abuse, drug dependence, epilepsy, chronic physical illness (especially chronic painful conditions), bereavement, social isolation, psychiatric disorder (apart from obsessional illness), family history of suicide or depression, previous suicide attempts and unemployment.

16 Schizophrenia   **Answers: B D**

Schizophrenia with an early onset usually results in a more chronic deterioration in personality. Affective change, such as depression, appears to indicate some preservation of personality and a better prognosis. Individual symptoms, such as visual hallucinations, do not appear to influence prognosis. Echolalia usually indicates an organic brain problem.

17 Multiple sclerosis   **Answers: B D**

Multiple sclerosis (MS) has a higher prevalence in temperate than in tropical countries. The Japanese have an exceptionally low incidence. MS may present with diplopia but it is due to involvement of cranial nerves III, IV or VI, not the optic nerve. MS quite frequently causes sensory disturbance of the limbs.

18 Bell's palsy   **Answers: B D E**

Dry eye caused by denervation of the lacrimal gland is very uncommon, whereas a watering eye is common. The salivary glands are not affected in Bell's palsy. Postauricular pain is common and may actually precede paralysis.

19 Nerves in the leg   Answers: A B E

In the arm, spasticity in a patient with hemiplegia is most pronounced in the flexor muscles and weakness in the extensor muscles. The converse is true in the leg. The peroneal nerve supplies skin over the lateral aspect of the lower leg. The saphenous branch of the femoral nerve supplies skin over the medial aspect of the lower leg. A femoral nerve palsy causes weakness of knee extension. A sciatic nerve palsy causes weakness of hip extension, knee flexion and foot dorsiflexion, plantarflexion, inversion and eversion.

20 Multiple sclerosis   Answers: B E

The diagnosis of multiple sclerosis (MS) is predominantly a clinical one, requiring discrete lesions in time and space. Investigations only aid in confirming your suspicion. Magnetic resonance imaging has become the investigation of choice. Visual-evoked potentials can be measured and are abnormal even in the absence of previous optic neuritis. Both hemianopia and dysphasia are extremely rare manifestations of MS. Epilepsy is more common, occurring in approximately 5% as a late complication. Red and green colour impairment or dimming of vision are common sequelae of optic neuritis. Bad prognostic signs are being male, onset after 40 years, predominant motor signs, poor recovery between each relapse and a short interval between each episode.

21 Stroke   Answers: A B

Stroke is more common in people in lower socioeconomic groups, probably because they smoke more and are more likely to suffer from hypertension. About 50% of patients with intracerebral or subarachnoid haemorrhage die within 30 days of their stroke, while in cerebral infarction the mortality is only 10%. Hypertension is the most important risk factor for stroke.

SINGLE BEST ANSWER QUESTIONS

1 Alzheimer's disease   **Answer: F**

Alzheimer's disease is the most common cause of dementia. Amnesia
and spatial dysfunction are typical early clinical features and social
graces are usually maintained until late in the disease. The underlying
pathology predominantly affects the temporal and parietal cortices.
Extrapyramidal rigidity, long tract signs and myoclonus are all late
clinical manifestations. The EEG is typically abnormal.

2 Differential diagnosis of dementia   **Answer: D**

The incidence of multi-infarct dementia varies greatly in different series.
This is undoubtedly due to the lack of a good differentiation test
between this and Alzheimer's disease. If a gait disturbance or urinary
incontinence appears early in the course of a dementing illness,
normal-pressure hydrocephalus should be considered. The presence of
any symptoms or signs which may arise from subcortical structures
should alert the clinician to diagnoses other than the pure cortical
dementias (eg Wilson's disease, Huntington's disease or Parkinson's
disease may need to be considered). The rapid progression of a
dementing process with associated long tract signs, myoclonic jerks and
severe rigidity point to the possibility of Creutzfeldt-Jakob disease. An
EEG is abnormal in approximately 90% of cases of Creutzfeldt-Jakob
disease, showing characteristic changes.

3 Alcohol   **Answer: B**

The relationship between alcohol and risk of death is complicated: the
lowest risk appears to be in those who consume 7–21 units per week. A
combination of a raised MCV and a raised gamma-GT will pick up
90% of problem drinkers. A similar proportion will answer 'yes' to two
of the five CAGE questions.

4   Risk of suicide   Answer: E

The most obvious warning sign of suicide is a direct statement of intent by the patient. There is no truth in the theory that people who talk about killing themselves actually do not do it. The presence of a feeling of hopelessness is a predictor of both immediate and subsequent suicide. Of the social factors, positive family history of suicide, prolonged physical illness and living alone indicate a higher risk. Paranoid delusions can occur in depressive illness, but do not have any special significance in assessing suicide risk.

5   Chronic fatigue syndrome   Answer: B

Few risk factors have been identified for chronic fatigue syndrome apart from previous psychiatric illness. More than 75% of affected patients have a concurrent psychiatric illness, depression being present in more than half. No relationship has been demonstrated between clinical status and any laboratory findings. The treatment of choice appears to be a structured return to physical activity and cognitive behavioural therapy, with treatment of any associated depression.

6   Tricyclic antidepressants   Answer: D

The tricyclic antidepressants have a number of important side-effects. They can produce dry mouth, blurred vision, urinary retention, constipation, postural hypotension, tachycardia and increased sweating. They can also cause fine tremor, inco-ordination, headaches, epileptic fits and peripheral neuropathy. Tricyclics are contraindicated in glaucoma. Tricyclic antidepressants may be used in patients with ischaemic heart disease, with caution. They are safe in patients anticoagulated with warfarin.

7   Post-herpetic neuralgia   Answer: D

Gabapentin and amitriptyline are both effective for post-herpetic neuralgia. Topical capsaicin is effective but may cause skin irritation. Epidural morphine is effective but not appropriate for the majority of patients.

8   Motor neurone disease   **Answer: A**

As the name motor neurone disease implies, degeneration occurs in the motor neurones. One group of motor neurones has its origin in the motor and pre-motor cortex, terminating in the brain stem or spinal cord. The second group has its origin in the brain stem or spinal cord, terminating in the muscle fibres.

9   Multiple sclerosis   **Answer: E**

Of the treatments mentioned, the only treatment proved to reduce the severity of relapse in multiple sclerosis is dietary supplementation with linoleic acid. Trials have shown both azathioprine and hyperbaric oxygen to be ineffective and potentially dangerous. Corticosteroids and ACTH bring forward remission following relapse but do not modify the overall course of the disease.

10 Migraine   **Answer: A**

Migraine without aura occurs in 75% of patients. Daily headaches are never migrainous. Although migrainous headaches are usually unilateral, they can occasionally be bilateral. Migrainous attacks are probably caused by the release of vasogenic amines from blood vessel walls accompanied by pulsatile distension.

11 Backache   **Answer: D**

Symptoms of nerve root irritation, such as unilateral leg pain worse than back pain and pain radiating to the buttocks, do not need specialist referral. Perineal anaesthesia, sphincter disturbance or gait disturbance are neurosurgical emergencies and require immediate referral. Presentation under 20 or over 55 may indicate malignancy and prompt referral (less than four weeks) should be considered. (RCGP guidelines.)

SUMMARY COMPLETION QUESTION

THEME: COELIAC DISEASE AND SCHIZOPHRENIA

1	H	(causation)
2	C	(association)
3	K	(homogeneous)
4	N	(inclusion)
5	I	(exclusion)
6	E	(under diagnosed)
7	F	(serological)
8	B	(converse)
9	M	(linkage)
10	D	(location)

SUMMARY COMPLETION QUESTION

THEME: GULF WAR ILLNESS

1	J	(cohort)
2	N	(randomly)
3	P	(comparable)
4	A	(outcome)
5	C	(heterogeneous)
6	Q	(subjective)
7	E	(standardised)
8	F	(confounder)

REPRODUCTIVE/RENAL

EXTENDED MATCHING QUESTIONS

THEME: COMMON CANCERS

1   **A**   Breast cancer

2   **A**   Breast cancer

3   **C**   Endometrial cancer

4   **D**   Ovarian cancer

5   **B**   Cervical cancer

6   **B**   Cervical cancer

Look carefully at clinical scenario questions for the hints that will give you the 'correct' answer. The most common malignant tumour that affects women only is breast cancer, which is also associated with an early menarche, rapid establishment of regular menstruation, obesity and high alcohol intake. Endometrial cancer is linked with unopposed oestrogen use and progestogen oral contraception may be protective. Ovarian cancer is more common in nulliparous and subfertile women, and sometimes has a familial tendency. Cervical cancer is linked with early teenage sexual intercourse, increased parity and smoking and has been linked to oral contraceptive use over more than 10 years.

THEME: MENSTRUAL DISTURBANCES

7   B   Cervical erosion

8   C   Climacteric

9   E   Fibroids

10   D   Endometriosis

11   I   Polycystic ovarian syndrome (PCOS)

12   G   Normal menstrual cycle

Cervical erosions occur at times of high oestrogen levels, such as pregnancy, puberty and when on the Pill. Non-offensive clear discharge and occasional post-coital spotting may occur. Cryocautery may be used if the discharge is troublesome. The climacteric is characterised by irregular cycles, hot flushes, intermittently heavy bleeds and mood changes. The mean age of onset in the UK is 51 (range 40–57). Fibroids are benign smooth muscle tumours, commoner in Africans and enlarge slowly in pregnancy and on the Pill. Symptoms are due to a mass effect (frequency and distension) and an increase in endometrial surface area (menorrhagia). Endometriosis is typically seen in 30- to 45-year-old women with dysmenorrhoea, menorrhagia, dyspareunia and infertility. PCOS classically causes infertility, obesity, hirsutism and menstrual disturbances. It can be diagnosed clinically, by ultrasound or with a raised LH/FSH ratio. The 'normal' intermenstrual interval of 28 days is only seen in 12% of women not on the Pill. Asking patients to keep a diary over three to four cycles will often confirm regular cycles.

THEME: CONTRACEPTION

13 H   Minipill

14 E   Implanon®

15 F   Intra-uterine device (IUD) insertion

16 B   Depo-Provera®

17 C   Diaphragm

18 I   Mirena® intra-uterine system

The combined pill is contraindicated in women over 35 who smoke and have high blood pressure. The minipill is the best choice in this situation as its effectiveness in terms of pregnancies in users per year is very good in older women. This will give her time to think about future options, eg sterilisation. A good choice here in travellers would be Implanon®. Starting the Pill now would not allow follow-up, and she is concerned about DVT. Depo-Provera® only lasts 12 weeks. Implanon® provides three years protection and is easily reversible. It does however require skilled insertion and removal. For emergency contraception, speed is of the essence. After 72 hours the only option is IUD insertion which may be done up to five days after intercourse. Focal migraine and ergotamine both preclude the use of oestrogenic contraceptives due to a risk of stroke. The minipill is not particularly effective in younger users and must be taken at the same time each day. Depo-Provera® is highly effective and easy to use. The diaphragm in combination with spermicide may be an effective choice for women approaching the menopause who still require contraception. Mirena® offers excellent contraception and the majority are amennorhoeic within six months. It works for five years.

MULTIPLE BEST ANSWER QUESTIONS

1 Postnatal depression

Answers: A B

Postnatal depression occurs in up to 25% of women after giving birth and is more common in women with a history of psychiatric illness. Surprisingly, women who have had obstetric complications do not seem to suffer more from postnatal depression. Suicide attempts by women shortly after birth are very rare. Antidepressant drugs are secreted only in small amounts into breast milk so treatment by them using moderate dosages is safe.

2 Breast-feeding

Answers: B C D

Human milk is low in protein compared with cows' milk, but cows' milk and human milk have similar fat contents. Hindmilk is more nutritious than foremilk, containing twice as much fat on average. Vitamin K levels in breast milk are low, which perhaps explains why haemorrhagic disease of the newborn is most common in breast-fed babies. An exclusively breast-fed infant will start becoming short of iron at about 6 months.

3 Chlamydia infections

Answers: C D

Chlamydia infections are found in about 5% of women attending General Practitioners. It is the commonest curable sexually transmitted disease (STD) in the developed world. Seventy-five per cent of cases seem to be asymptomatic but long-term effects are infertility and ectopic pregnancy. Screening can be difficult but it appears to be possible using urine samples.

4 Carcinoma of the cervix

Answers: A B

There has been a large increase in the number of women having cervical smears and a steady fall in both incidence and mortality from cervical cancer. Human papillomavirus (HPV) is sexually transmitted and a strong link with cervical cancer exists, in that almost all cases of cervical cancer have HPV infection. However, most women with HPV infection will not develop cancer of the cervix.

5   Contraception   Answers: A B C D

The Pill has many positive advantages in addition to its contraceptive effect. It suppresses both benign breast disease and ovarian cysts. It also decreases the rate of pelvic inflammatory disease and the risk of ovarian cancer. However, use of the Pill does increase the risk of pulmonary embolism, arterial disease and possibly increases the risk of breast cancer.

6   Hormonal post-coital contraception   Answers: B E

A short course of high-dose progestogen is more reliable as post-coital contraception than a mixture of oestrogen and progestogen. The first dose is taken as soon as possible after unprotected intercourse, the second dose 12 hours later. It can be up to 72 hours but has greater efficacy if taken soon after unprotected intercourse. If there is any vomiting, the dose should be repeated immediately. One should exclude pregnancy if periods are delayed.

7   Antenatal women   Answers: A C E

Women are best advised to take folic acid from pre-conception and for the first trimester – 5 mg a day if a previous baby had neural tube defects and 0.4 mg for others. Increased vitamins from diet are usually sufficient and the addition of multivitamin supplements has little effect. Moreover, vitamin A in high doses can be teratogenic. Giving all pregnant women iron supplements is not advised unless the mother has true iron deficiency. Soft ripened cheeses such as Brie and Camembert should not be eaten during pregnancy; hard cheeses can be eaten. Pâtés may be contaminated with *Listeria*.

8   Causes of menorrhagia   Answers: B C D

Causes also include polyps, endometrial cancer, dysfunctional uterine bleeding, endometriosis and blood dyscrasias. Psychological causes can be implicated as the perception of blood loss is very subjective. Myxoedema rather than thyrotoxicosis is associated with menorrhagia. Fibroids can be associated with menorrhagia, presumably due to the increased surface area of the endometrium. The IUCD causes direct effects that result in menorrhagia. Anorexia and thyrotoxicosis usually cause amenorrhoea.

9   Pre-eclampsia   Answers: A C D

Predisposition to pre-eclampsia occurs in diabetics, primigravida and twin pregnancies (possibly due to the large placenta). Hydatidiform moles are associated with an increased incidence of pre-eclampsia.

10 Contraception counselling   Answers: B C

The Gillick ruling allowed doctors to provide contraception legally to girls under 16, without parental consent. It is not always essential to take a full sexual history, but important facts need to be established and realisation of under-age sex needs to be kept in mind. It is not recommended to use an IUCD or Mirena®.

11 Puerperal psychosis   Answers: B E F

Puerperal psychosis usually begins within the first two weeks. There are three main types of clinical picture: acute organic, affective (depressive or manic) and schizophrenic. The most common presentation is depressive. The onset is usually acute and the prognosis good. The risk of recurrence in subsequent pregnancies is between 1:3 and 1:7.

12 Perimenopausal contraception   Answers: B D

FSH levels are reliable in progesterone-only pill users, but not in combined pill users. The IUCD is a possibility, including Mirena®.

13 Puerperal psychosis   Answers: B C D

The majority of puerperal psychoses begin within the first two weeks after childbirth, and rarely in the first two days. The illness usually starts with a period of delirium. The outlook is favourable. Auditory hallucinations are frequently experienced, but obsessional ruminations are not part of the clinical picture.

14 Torsion of the testis   Answers: A B D

Torsion of the testis is most common in the 12–22 years age group, generally after a physical injury, usually from sport. It usually presents with abdominal pain and vomiting and always requires urgent referral, as delay can lead to a non-viable testis. At operation, if the testis is non-viable it should always be removed, as antibodies will cause infertility. An average General Practitioner is more than likely to see at least one case in their lifetime.

15 Benign prostatic hypertrophy (BPH)   Answers: A C

The prevalence of BPH is increasing as the population is ageing and more patients are reporting symptoms. Nocturia is a very poor diagnostic feature, as this can have several causes including insomnia, or large fluid intake. Beta-blockers remain drugs of choice, despite the fact that they do not reduce the size of the prostate gland. The number of transurethral prostatectomies has more than halved in the last ten years. PSA test should only be offered to patients after careful counselling in selected groups.

16 Prostatic cancer   Answers: A D

Prostatic cancer is usually an adenocarcinoma and all types of tumour are found from well differentiated to poorly differentiated. This range of differentiation may even be seen within the same tumour. Prostate-specific antigen is an accurate marker of prostate cancer but not a reliable diagnostic investigation because it can be raised in patients with benign hypertrophy. Prostate cancer responds objectively to hormone therapy in about 40% of cases.

SINGLE BEST ANSWER QUESTIONS

1 Prostate cancer   Answer: D

PSA testing does not fulfil all of Wilson's criteria for screening. The National Screening Committee currently advises against screening for prostate cancer. PSA has a poor specificity, but is readily available. Some of the prostate cancers detected by screening would never present clinically, and the prostate biopsies may indeed cause some harm. PSA cannot predict whether a cancer is in a dormant or aggressive form.

2 Childhood urinary tract infection   Answer: E

Although most children come to no harm from urinary tract infection (UTI) the fundamental objective is to identify those at risk of developing permanent renal damage. Diagnosis of UTI usually requires pure urinary culture of 10^5 bacteria per ml. Childhood UTI is associated with vesico-ureteric reflux in two out of three affected children and is caused by an unsuspected surgical disorder in 5% of children. Single antibiotics are usually used for treatment, for example trimethoprim.

3 Breast cancer   Answer: C

Breast cancer is the most common cancer affecting women, with every woman having about a 1 in 10 risk of developing breast cancer in her life. Screening women over 50 years of age may produce a decrease in mortality. Extending the age range of women in the screening programme from 65 to 70 may prevent more deaths. However, shortening the interval from three to two years between screening sessions may gain more life-years. Tamoxifen treatment improves survival by 15–20% with oestrogen-receptor-positive tumours. Tamoxifen also reduces the incidence of cancer in the other breast. However, the risk of endometrial cancer appears to be increased.

4 Oral contraceptive steroids   Answer: C

Oral contraceptive steroids protect against benign breast disease and carcinoma of the uterus and ovary. The risk of venous thrombosis and pulmonary embolism is related to the oestrogen content of the combined contraceptive pill.

5   Endometrial cancer   Answer: D

Progestogen-based oral contraceptives may have a protective effect against endometrial cancer. Endometrial cancer is usually a well-differentiated adenocarcinoma.

6   Oral contraceptive pill   Answer: D

There is no evidence that progesterone alone increases blood pressure. Even in low dose, the combined oestrogen and progesterone contraceptive pill increases arterial pressure. Established or developing hypertension is therefore a contraindication to a combined pill. Oestrogens increase the risk of arterial or venous thrombosis in some women. The progesterone-only preparation appears safe. If a women of over 35 years smokes, then the risk of serious cardiovascular events is greatly elevated if she is receiving a combined, but not a progesterone-only, pill. Certain tumours may be oestrogen sensitive, eg malignant melanoma, hepatoma, desmoid tumours or carcinoma of the breast. As with oestrogens, the metabolism of progesterone is increased by the concurrent use of anticonvulsants that are hepatic enzyme inducers. The combined preparations probably do not enhance the risk of thrombotic crises in sickle cell disease.

7   Bladder cancer   Answer: C

Bladder cancer is usually a transitional cell carcinoma. Most tumours at presentation are superficial. Up to 30% of superficial tumours become invasive, despite adequate treatment. Chemotherapy for metastases improves life expectancy.

8   Prostate cancer   Answer: E

Prostate cancer is the most common cancer in men, and the second commonest cause of cancer death after lung cancer. Over 50% have metastatic spread at diagnosis. Pain is a common feature in the terminal care. Screening results in greatly increased detection but without clear indication of improved survival.

SUMMARY COMPLETION QUESTION

THEME: ORAL CONTRACEPTIVE USE

1	**E**	(incidence)
2	**G**	(indicative)
3	**N**	(dispensing)
4	**A**	(prescribing)
5	**P**	(compliance)
6	**K**	(increased)
7	**O**	(numerator)
8	**B**	(denominator)

RESPIRATORY MEDICINE

EXTENDED MATCHING QUESTIONS

THEME: BREATHLESSNESS

1   A   Allergic alveolitis

2   D   Lung cancer

3   B   Asthma

4   F   Pulmonary embolism

5   E   Myocardial infarction

In clinical scenarios look carefully at the whole scenario searching for key features. Decide on the diagnosis and then look to see if it is in the option list. Look again now at these scenarios with the 'correct' answers in mind. Notice the aviary in the history and the crepitations in the examination of the patient with allergic alveolitis. The female sex, younger age and use of oral contraceptives make a diagnosis of pulmonary embolism more likely in the fourth patient.

THEME: BREATHLESSNESS

6   K   Pulmonary fibrosis

7   H   Pleural effusion

8   A   Anaemia

9   I   Pneumothorax

10 E   Inhalation of foreign body

11 G   Left ventricular failure

Pulmonary fibrosis may be secondary to inhalation of dust or chemicals, idiopathic, iatrogenic (eg after radiotherapy), congenital or a pulmonary manifestation of systemic disease, eg rheumatoid arthritis. Pleural effusion may be caused by many conditions, including ovarian hyperstimulation syndrome, where it is associated with ascites. Breathlessness may be caused by disease of the lungs and heart, but extrathoracic causes should always be considered as well. Expansion of trapped air in the alveolar tree on ascent may cause alveolar rupture and pneumothorax in scuba divers. This may lead to cerebral arterial gas embolism. For this reason asthmatics (who often have a degree of air trapping) and patients with a history of spontaneous pneumothorax should not dive. Inhalation of foreign bodies may also present subacutely with signs of localised rhonchi and crepitations if smaller objects pass into the lower bronchi. Left ventricular failure may be precipitated by myocardial infarction, arrhythmias or fluid overload.

MULTIPLE BEST ANSWER QUESTIONS

1 Childhood asthma   Answers: A B

Cough may be the only symptom in some children. Outdoor exercise should not be discouraged. Inhaled steroids are usually used for prevention – they do not normally stunt growth. Sodium chromoglycate can be used but is not the drug of choice.

2 Smoking   Answers: A C

GP advice is effective in helping smoking cessation. Nicotine replacement therapy appears to double the rate of smoking cessation achieved by GP advice alone. Many patients will have already thought about their smoking habit and the doctor–patient relationship can be harmed if routine anti-smoking advice is given to all patients. The current increase in smoking is due to the number of younger people starting to smoke. People who have never smoked have a much greater risk of ischaemic heart disease if they live with a smoker.

3 Severe asthma attack   Answers: A C D

Severe asthma is characterised by frequent attacks, limited daily activities, disturbed sleep to 'early morning dips', low PEFR readings (usually 50% or less of normal PEFR readings) and tachycardia. Central cyanosis rather than peripheral cyanosis occurs in severe asthma.

4 Chronic obstructive pulmonary disease   Answers: A C

After standardisation for smoking, men are still more at risk than women for chronic obstructive pulmonary disease. Low socioeconomic status is also a risk factor.

5 Lung cancer   Answers: A B E

Lung cancer is most prevalent among people aged over 70 years and causes deaths in the ratio 2:1, men to women, in the UK. It is associated with the level of urban pollution. Adenocarcinoma occurs amongst non-smokers and squamous cell carcinoma among smokers. No genetic association has been clearly established for lung cancer.

6   Increased resonance   **Answers: B C D**

In pneumothorax and emphysema, the liver may be pushed downwards
to give the impression of hepatomegaly.

SINGLE BEST ANSWER QUESTIONS

1 British Thoracic Society guidelines for asthma   **Answer: B**

The British Thoracic Society guidelines for asthma indicate that inhaled short acting beta-agonist should be given as required as the first step; if inhaled short acting beta-agonists are needed more than once a day an inhaled steroid should be used. Step three involves the addition of a long acting beta agonist. Step four involves the consideration of increased inhaled steroid use or theophylline or a beta-agonist tablet.

2 Finger clubbing   **Answer: B**

Think of pulmonary (bronchiectasis, lung abscess, lung cancer), cardiac (cyanotic congenital heart disease, infective endocarditis) and extrathoracic (cirrhosis, inflammatory bowel disease) causes. It occurs in empyema rather than emphysema.

3 Inhaled steroids   **Answer: B**

Some systemic absorption will take place. Inhaled steroid in high dosage may slow growth in children, but side-effects are unusual at low doses. Inhaled steroids are not indicated for use in episodic wheezing. Fluticasone may be less systemically absorbed.

4 Chest infections   **Answer: C**

Very few chest infections seen in General Practice are due to pneumonia, but the vast majority of patients with lower respiratory tract infections will receive antibiotics. Antibiotics are of value in an exacerbation of chronic obstructive pulmonary disease.

5 Asthma in children   **Answer: D**

Skin allergy tests are generally uninformative and should not be ordered routinely. Chest radiographs are only indicated for acute episodes if complications are suspected. Pulmonary function tests become reliable in children aged 7–8 years and over.

6   Recognised causes of cough   **Answer: C**

Common causes of cough include infections (upper and lower
respiratory), postnasal drip, asthma, smoking, lung cancer, inhaled
foreign body (especially peanuts), lung diseases (eg cystic fibrosis,
fibrosing alveolitis) and gastro-oesophageal reflux disease. Consider also
medication (ACE inhibitors due to effects on the bradykinin system in
the throat), pulmonary oedema ('cardiac asthma'), pertussis and TB.

7   Diagnosis of asthma   **Answer: B**

Cough is an essential feature in diagnosis and so is family history. The
reversibility test is useful, but not essential. Fifty per cent of children
with asthma are not asthmatic after the age of 7. Steroid inhalers do not
have an immediate effect and are for prevention.

8   Bronchial carcinoma   **Answer: E**

Bronchial carcinoma is now the most common malignant disease in
Western Europe. Occupational risk factors include exposure to asbestos,
nickel, arsenic, haematite, chromates and radioactivity.

9   Asthma   **Answer: D**

Asthma mortality has not improved significantly over the past 50 years.
Long-acting inhaled bronchodilators are usually recommended when
inhaled steroids have provided inadequate control. Viral infections
commonly precipitate attacks. Virtually all symptomatic asthmatics have
hyper-reactive airways, as do a significant number of the normal
population. There is no direct adrenergic innervation of the airways.
Beta-2 agonists act on adrenergic receptors.

PHOTO QUESTION

THEME: RESPIRATORY MEDICINE

1 B

This patient developed a cough on a cruise and rapidly deteriorated. The chest X-ray shows signs of lower respiratory tract infection. His symptoms settled with clarithromycin.

2 D

The spirometry results show a reduction in FEV1 with a normal FVC. This is often seen in asthma or chronic obstructive pulmonary disease.

3 A

This image shows clubbed fingers. In this case the history is suggestive of lung cancer, clubbing is often seen in this condition.

4 E

This history combined with reduced FEV1 and FVC suggests pulmonary fibrosis. Most cases are due to occupational exposure

5 C

This image shows erythema nodosum which may be associated with mycobacterial and streptococcal infections, drugs and inflammatory bowel disease. This patient had sarcoidosis, which affects the lungs in <90% of cases, characteristically with hilar lymphadenopathy, alveolitis or interstitial pneumonitis.

SUMMARY COMPLETION QUESTION

THEME: CHEST PAIN CLINIC

1	F	(dilemma)
2	H	(maximise)
3	C	(minimise)
4	N	(triaged)
5	P	(supernumerary)
6	E	(placebo effects)
7	A	(health seeking behaviour)
8	Q	(significant)
9	D	(insignificant)
10	L	(do not)

SUMMARY COMPLETION QUESTION

THEME: COPD SCREENING

1	D	(applicability)
2	G	(vital)
3	A	(socioeconomically)
4	I	(morbidity)
5	C	(pro-active)
6	K	(opportunity cost)
7	E	(tiotropium)
8	H	(targeted)
9	F	(outcome)
10	B	(smoking cessation)

SUMMARY COMPLETION QUESTION

THEME: OVER-THE-COUNTER REMEDIES

1 **I**   (working hypotheses)

2 **E**   (qualitative)

3 **L**   (pilot)

4 **C**   (underpowered)

5 **J**   (extrapolation)

6 **A**   (bias)

7 **O**   (representative)

8 **G**   (post hoc)

9 **M**   (natural history)

10 **Q**   (methodology)

ADMINISTRATION AND
MANAGEMENT ANSWERS

ADMINISTRATION AND MANAGEMENT ANSWERS

EXTENDED MATCHING QUESTIONS

THEME: CONSULTATION: WRITERS, MODELS AND THEORIES

1   C   Berne

2   E   Heron

3   A   Biomedical Model

4   I   Stott and Davis

5   A   Biomedical Model

6   G   Pendleton, Schofield, Tate and Havelock

7   D   Byrne and Long

You should aim to know about several models of consultation. The Biomedical model involves the classical medical diagnostic process; it relies on an objective medical disorder being found, and does not consider the doctor–patient relationship. Berne identified three ego states, parent, adult, and child. Heron described six types intervention: prescriptive, informative, confronting, cathartic, catalytic and supportive. Stott and Davis mentioned a four-pronged approach involving management of presenting and continuing problems, as well as changing help-seeking behaviour and opportunistic health promotion. Byrne and Long used the terms doctor-centred and patient-centred, and analysed thousands of tape-recorded consultations. Pendleton, Schofield, Tate and Havelock's model described seven stages or tasks in a consultation and could involve consultation mapping.

THEME: LEGISLATION

8 **E** Rehabilitation of Offenders Act 1974

9 **B** Access to Medical Reports Act 1988

10 **A** Access to Health Records Act 1990

11 **D** Disability Discrimination Act 1995

12 **C** Data Protection Act 1984

You need to know some of the background about these Acts:

- Data Protection Act 1984 – controls computer-held personal data

- Rehabilitation of Offenders Act 1974 – results in certain convictions being 'spent'

- Disability Discrimination Act 1995 – gives employers duties in relation to employees with present or past disabilities

- Access to Health Records Act 1990 – allows patients access to their own medical notes

- Access to Medical Reports Act 1988 – allows patients to see reports

THEME: VOLUNTARY ORGANISATIONS

13 J   RNIB

14 D   CRUSE

15 I   RELATE

16 G   MIND

17 M   Terrence Higgins Trust

18 C   Compassionate Friends

19 A   Alanon

20 H   NSPCC

21 E   Gingerbread

22 F   Marie Curie Memorial Foundation

23 D   CRUSE

24 B   ASH

25 N   Turning point

There are many voluntary organisations. You should at least know what
they are concerned with:

- RNIB – blindness
- CRUSE – widows with bereavement problems and children
  suffering bereavement problems after death of parents
- RELATE – marriage problems
- MIND – mental illness
- Terrence Higgins Trust – AIDS
- Compassionate Friends – bereaved parents
- Alanon – relatives of people with alcohol problems
- NSPCC – child abuse
- Gingerbread – one parent families
- Marie Curie Memorial Foundation – cancer
- ASH – smokers
- Turning Point – drug abuse

THEME: MEDICAL CERTIFICATES

26 D   Med 6

27 A   Med 3

28 D   Med 6̶ 10

29 F   DS 1500

30 B   Med 4

31 A   Med 3

32 C   Med 5

All medical practitioners must know about certification for sickness absence. Med 3 is the usual sickness certificate – the patient must be seen, and this certificate can initially be issued for up to six months. Med 4 is only issued when the personal capability incapacity test is being considered. Med 5 is issued when a patient was seen previously or there is a recent medical report about the patient. Med 6 is to be used when a vague diagnosis has deliberately been put on another certificate – usually in the interests of confidentiality. Hospital personnel issue Med 10. A DS 1500 is issued when a patient has a terminal illness and has applied for Disability Living Allowance or Attendance Allowance.

THEME: NUMBERS OF PEOPLE ON A GP'S LIST

33 E   100

34 A   5

35 C   25

36 F   200

37 B   10

You need to have a good idea about the frequency of events and the occurrence of diseases. In an average GP list, there will be 5 schizophrenics, 10 blind people, 25 deaf people, 100 unemployed people and 200 people on state benefits.

MULTIPLE BEST ANSWER QUESTIONS

1   Learning profile   **Answers: C D**

A learning portfolio is a record of past experience of learning and gives future plans. The portfolio could include audit, research projects and patient surveys.

2   GPs complaints procedure   **Answers: A C**

All GPs must operate a practice-based complaints procedure and the procedure must be practice owned. All staff must support the procedure. The complaints procedure must be adequately publicised with detailed written information.

3   Competency   **Answers: D E**

A competent adult can refuse treatment if the treatment is indicated even if death would result or it would be detrimental to a fetus. To be competent the person needs to retain information long enough to allow an effective decision, and understand the nature and purpose of treatment, including the risks, benefits and the alternatives.

4   Consultation by email   **Answers: C D**

Consulting by email can be used to help book appointments, and it is possible that patients might make contact from abroad. It is thought that email consultations are likely to increase workload. They would not avoid problems with GMC and medical defence organisations, and are not generally encouraged by the GMC and GP committees.

5   New contract of 2003   **Answers: B C**

In the new contract of 2003 the contract is between the practice and PCT. All practices must provide health care to all who believe themselves to be ill. There are also directed enhanced services and the care of violent patients is one such service. Minor surgery is also a directed enhanced service, but cryosurgery is considered to be an additional service (services that most GPs provide). Contraceptive services are another example of an additional service.

6   Revalidation   Answers: C D

It is expected that the vast majority of doctors will be recommended for revalidation. Revalidation applies to all doctors on the current register. It involves the demonstration of good clinical care and requires doctors to sign declarations about their own health and probity. Revalidation is seen as a collection of information with a yearly appraisal and 5-yearly assessment with a GMC decision.

7   Independent contractor status of GPs   Answers: B C

There are questions with negatives in the stem and then in one or more items, so make sure that you read such questions carefully! It might be easier to think, in this question, about arguments in favour of the independent contractor status of GPs, and then reverse those options.

The independent contractor status of GPs allows a flexible working pattern, allows GPs greater control of their jobs, eg staffing levels, and allows them to act independently on behalf of patients. Unfortunately money can be a concern and doctors certainly do need to listen to the PCTs and follow NSFs.

8   Consent for a child   Answers: B C

Consent for children can be given by a child's mother if not married at the time of conception or birth, but not by a child's father if he was not married to the mother at the time of conception or birth. Consent can be given by person holding a residence order from a court, or a local authority designated in a court order.

9   Seizures   Answers: A D E

The patient, but not his or her doctor, is obliged to contact the DVLA, although it is sensible practice to record in the case notes that a patient has been counselled about driving. Patients must be free from any attack for two years, or have had only attacks whilst asleep for three years, before driving is permitted. A diagnosis of primary malignant cerebral tumour, cerebral metastasis or even bronchogenic carcinoma without cerebral metastasis is associated with such a high risk of a seizure that driving is prohibited.

10 History of epilepsy   Answers: B C

Teachers in training have to have been seizure-free for two years. Similarly, a recent history would be a problem for a prison officer. Any history of epilepsy would be a barrier for employment as aircraft pilots, train drivers and army officers. Merchant seafarers must not have had a fit since the age of 5 years.

11 Burnout in General Practitioners   Answers: B D E

Burnout appears to be a response to stress and dissatisfaction. There is a relation to depressive illness. Obsessional, idealistic and conscientious doctors, who are reluctant to delegate, are more likely to get burnt out. Fortunately, attendance at postgraduate meetings and postgraduate qualifications seem to have a protective influence against burnout.

12 Heartsink patients   Answers: C D E

Postgraduate qualifications and counselling training appear to reduce the number of patients seen or perceived as heartsink patients. Lower job satisfaction and a greater number of heartsink patients are related, but it is unclear which is cause or effect. About one-third have a serious medical diagnosis of some sort and non-attendance at appointments is high.

13 Over-the-counter medicines   Answers: A C D

Medicines should be POM if they are normally administered by injection, if they are new and need further investigation, if they are frequently used incorrectly and if they are dangerous if used other than under medical supervision. Cimetidine has been over-the-counter (OTC) since 1993 while ibuprofen has been available since 1983 and topical aciclovir since 1993. Piroxicam is available OTC only in topical form (since 1994).

14 Free NHS prescriptions   Answers: B D E

Patients with myxoedema or conditions requiring supplemental thyroxine get free prescriptions, as do some thyrotoxics needing concomitant thyroxine. Diabetics on diet alone do not get free prescriptions. Free prescriptions are available to patients with a permanent fistula, eg caecostomy, colostomy, laryngostomy or ileostomy, needing continuous surgical dressing or appliance, and for patients with hypoparathyroidism, hypopituitarism or continuing physical disability needing the help of another person. Don't forget free prescriptions for pregnant women.

15 Advance directives   Answers: B C D

An advance directive can be revoked if the patient requests this and is competent to make that request. There is a need to be explicit about the possibility of death in the directive, which needs to be signed and witnessed. The advance directive must not be deliberately ignored. Very basic care, including hydration and nutrition, will be maintained.

16 Confirmation of death   Answers: A B E

Reportable deaths are where the cause is unknown, unnatural cause, abortion, suicide, industrial disease, due to medication, drugs or poisons, deaths due to injury, not seen by a medical practitioner in the last illness or not seen in the last 14 days.

17 Prescription on FP10   Answers: A B D

Viagra® can be prescribed in a limited group; patients outside this category can only be given private treatment. Paracetamol can be given, but not as Panadol®. Neck collars can be obtained from hospitals, but not on FP10.

18 Patient records   Answers: C E

Paper records are the property of the Secretary of State. A patient may include a statement contesting the report but may not insist on it being amended. Third party details may be disguised to protect individuals. Practices may make a reasonable charge for access to any records.

SINGLE BEST ANSWER QUESTIONS

1   PMS   Answer: E

PMS was set up to attract GPs to areas of recruitment problems, to tackle inequalities of health, and to get GPs and nurses working more closely with joint or shared responsibility. There is no single national contract; instead all practices have an individual contract negotiated with the PCT. The budgets for PMS are not guaranteed, and the independent role of GPs is threatened.

2   Training practices   Answer: B

When a practice becomes a training practice the patients should be informed, perhaps in the practice leaflet. The issue about workload for the partners is not clear: it is likely to increase initially. The partners' views on organisational matters are likely to be challenged by the registrar, who should not be excluded from all practice meetings. The practice is expected to organise any special equipment (eg video) that is needed by the registrar or trainer.

3   New contract of 2003   Answer: C

Following the new contract of 2003, all practices will receive a global sum and extra money for quality payments. The Carr Hill formula is used to calculate the global sum, which is for essential, additional and enhanced services. There are six quality domains which include clinical and organisational aspects; quality payments are not made via the PCT.

4   Self-regulation   Answer: B

In self-regulation the profession decides on its own codes of ethics and behaviour. It may be more difficult with a better-informed public and is threatened by loss of public confidence. Self-regulation might be perceived in allowing the profession to protect its own interests, but the profession must demonstrate that this is not the case.

5   New contract of 2003   Answer: A

The new contract for GPs means that it is possible to opt out of 24-hour responsibility, seniority payments start earlier, PCT will purchase all IT equipment, and pensions will improve. There is more flexibility with a greater number of salaried positions.

6   Personal Development Plans   Answer: E

Personal Development Plans require learning portfolios for all members of the practice team, and combine personal self-directed learning with an organisational development framework

7   Commercial flights   Answer: B

Most commercial flights will allow pregnant women of up to 34 weeks' gestational age to be carried on board.

8   Mental Health Act 1983   Answer: B

Section 3 is the most appropriate section to use for a patient with an established psychiatric diagnosis who has to be admitted compulsorily for treatment.

9   General Medical Council   Answer: C

The General Medical Council has recently revised its guidance to doctors and these are published as five separate booklets. Most of the information is covered under *Duties of the Doctor*. Doctors do not have to meet performance targets set by management if they disagree with them, but if non-provision of the targets can be shown to cause harm to patients, the doctor would have a very weak case.

10 Complaints   Answer: E

There must be a nominated person and a deputy to administer the system, but these may be anyone in the practice. An acknowledgement must be made within two working days and a response within 10. The time limit to lodge a complaint is one year. Ninety per cent of complaints are due to failure to visit, examine, diagnose or refer.

RESEARCH, EPIDEMIOLOGY AND STATISTICS

RESEARCH, EPIDEMIOLOGY AND STATISTICS

EXTENDED MATCHING QUESTIONS

THEME: ORLISTAT

1	K	30
2	J	28
3	T	Hypertension
4	C	2.5
5	P	Dietary
6	R	Activity
7	E	5
8	F	6
9	G	10
10	A	1
11	B	2

Orlistat (Xenical®) is a pancreatic lipase inhibitor. It helps weight loss by impairing uptake of fats in the gut. It has no effect on uptake of calories in any other form, so patients must lose weight by a reduction in calorie intake. It may lead to faecal incontinence if fats are consumed and potentially may lead to a deficiency of the fat-soluble vitamins A, D, E and K.

THEME: STATISTICS

12 B   112/175

13 A   112/183

14 J   754/817

15 K   754/825

However, the way the question is presented, it is best to write out the figures in a table:

	Disease present	Disease absent	Total
Test positive	112	71	183
Test negative	63	754	817
Total	175	825	1000

Then:

Sensitivity = 112/175

Specificity = 754/825

Positive predictive value = 112/183

Negative predictive value = 754/817

THEME: TRIALS

16 D   Descriptive study

17 A   Case–control study

18 F   Randomised clinical trial

19 C   Correlation study

20 E   Meta-analysis study

You need to be clear about the types of trials and studies. Remember that:

- Cohort studies follow forward groups, otherwise matched, with different exposures to the topic of concern
- Case–control studies compare patients with the disease/problem with controls, looking at past exposure/events
- Correlation studies look for an association between quantitative variables.

THEME: STATISTICAL TERMS

21 E   2

22 E   2

23 E   2

It is best to put the numbers in order: 0, 0, 1, 1, 1, 2, 2, 2, 2, 4, 7.

The average (mean) is 22/11 = 2.

The median (in the middle) is 2.

The mode (most common) is 2.

THEME: ECONOMICS

24 B   Cost-benefit analysis

25 A   Cost

26 F   Cost-effectiveness ratio

27 H   Cost-of-illness analysis

28 I   Cost-utility analysis

A cost-benefit analysis is a type of economic assessment in which both cost and benefit are expressed in monetary terms. Cost is the monetary value of the resources consumed in production or delivery. The cost-effectiveness ratio is the ratio of total cost of an intervention divided by the gain in selected health outcome. Cost-of-illness analysis estimates the economic burden of a particular disease. Cost-utility analysis assesses the benefit of an intervention.

THEME: STUDIES

29 B   Cohort study

30 F   Randomised double-blind crossover trial

31 G   Randomised double-blind placebo-controlled trial

32 A   Case–control study

33 D   Descriptive study

Think about the types of trials and studies. Remember that:

Cohort studies are prospective studies following matched groups with different exposures to the subject of concern. Case–control studies are retrospective studies comparing patients with the disease/problem with controls and looking at past exposure/events. Correlation studies look for an association between quantitative variables. Descriptive studies often simply describe what has been found, or what prevalence of a disease has been noted.

THEME: SCREENING TESTS

34 H 80%

35 I 93%

36 D 25%

37 B 0.8

38 C 20%

	Disease	No disease
Test positive	*a* (20)	*b* (5)
Test negative	*c* (5)	*d* (70)

Sensitivity: a sensitive test detects a high proportion of the true cases, measured here by $a/(a + c)$

Specificity: a highly specific test has very few false positives, measured by $d/(b + d)$

Systematic error: this is measured by the ratio of the total numbers positive to the test and those with the disease, or $(a + b)/(a + c)$

Prevalence: $a + c/(a + b + c + d)$

Predictive value: this is the proportion of positive test results that are truly positive, measured as $a/(a + b)$. It is important in screening

Yield: $a/(a + b + c + d)$

Systematic error, yield and predictive value depend on the relative frequency of true positives and true negatives in the study sample (ie on the prevalence of the disease or exposure that is being measured).

THEME: RESEARCH METHODS

39 **A** Clinical audit

40 **F** Survey

41 **D** Qualitative study

42 **E** Randomised controlled trial

43 **B** Longitudinal study

These are examples of research methods now used in General Practice. The explanation is generally in the answer. Other studies may be used for some of the answers, but only the most likely answers are expected.

THEME: STATISTICAL TERMS

44 **B** Sensitivity analysis

45 **E** Standard deviation

46 **A** Sensitivity

47 **F** Standard error of the mean (SEM)

48 **H** Standardised mortality rate

Common definitions to common terms used in research papers. There is an expectation that you are familiar with these terms.

THEME: LITERATURE IN GENERAL PRACTICE

49 **F** Pendleton D

50 **G** Stott CP, Davis RH

51 **C** Byrne PS, Long BEL

52 **A** Balint M

53 **F** Pendleton D

54 **B** Berne E

55 **D** Heron J

56 **G** Stott CP, Davis RH

57 **E** Neighbour R

58 **A** Balint M

You need to be familiar with General Practice literature. Pendleton's *The Consultation* discusses seven tests and achieving a shared understanding with the patient. Balint's *The Doctor, his Patient and the Illness* describes both the apostolic function of the doctor, and the use of the doctor as a 'drug'.

THEME: A YEAR IN GENERAL PRACTICE

59 **E** <1

60 **A** 500

61 **B** 200

62 **D** 10

63 **C** 25

You need to have a good idea about the frequency of events and the occurrence of diseases. In an average year in an average General Practice, about 500 people consult because of chronic mental illness, about 200 because of hypertension, about 25 because of diabetes, about 10 with a thyroid problem, and less than 1 with chronic renal failure.

THEME: TRIALS CONCERNING CORONARY HEART DISEASE

64 D   GISSI

65 E   GREAT Group Study

66 A   4S

67 C   CARE Study

68 F   ISIS-2

69 G   Nurses Study

70 B   ASSET

Important trials of thrombolytic therapy include ISIS-2, GISSI and ASSET. ISIS-2 involved treating patients with streptokinase and/or aspirin. GISSI involved streptokinase and placebo. ASSET used alteplase.

The GREAT Group Study was about the pre-hospital treatment of patients using anistreplase as the active drug.

Two large-scale drug trials using lipid-lowering drugs on people needing secondary prevention were 4S and CARE Study. 4S used simvastatin; CARE used pravastatin therapy. The Nurses Study of unopposed oestrogen showed a large reduction in the incidence of ischaemic heart disease.

THEME: CARDIOVASCULAR TRIALS

71 I   WOSCOPS

72 G   SOLVD-T

73 C   CARE

74 F   ISIS-2

75 E   HOT

76 H   UKPDS-1998

The HOT trial confirmed that the lowest incidence of cardiovascular complications occurred at a diastolic BP of 82.6 mmHg. 4S looked at secondary prevention in patients with hypercholesterolaemia. HOPE confirmed the value of ramipril in high-risk patients. The Antiplatelet Trialists' Collaboration 94 demonstrated the benefit of aspirin 75 mg a day for secondary prevention. UKPDS-1998 in particular demonstrated the value of tight BP control in diabetes mellitus but also confirmed the value of metformin.

THEME: HYPERTENSION

77 **Q** Non-pharmacological measures

78 **G** 100

79 **C** 15

80 **I** 145

81 **D** 85

82 **J** 150

83 **E** 90

84 **T** Thiazides

85 **N** Beta-blockers

86 **M** Aspirin

87 **S** Statins

The general principles of the management of hypertension are to confirm the diagnosis with at least three separate readings, try lifestyle measures first, such as weight loss and exercise, then start treatment with low-dose thiazides or beta-blockers. The choice of second-line agent will depend on the patient: diabetics should be treated with ACE inhibitors, but these are relatively ineffective in black people and in the elderly. The full guidance can be found at www.hyp.ac.uk.

MULTIPLE BEST ANSWER QUESTIONS

1 Mental health of children and adolescents   Answers: A D E

Ten per cent of children between 5 and 15 years have a significant
mental disorder, with boys being particularly affected. Children in
families without a working parent are particularly vulnerable in this
respect. Almost 50% of children with a mental disorder will have been
seen by their GP that year but 30% have no contact with a GP or
specialist service. The proportion of children with special educational
needs is three times higher in children with a mental disorder.

2 Children   Answers: A D

Infant mortality in social class V is very much higher than that in social
class I. Children in social class V are more likely to die in an accident;
they have twice the rate of chronic illness and they are shorter.

3 Obesity in the UK   Answers: A E

The prevalence of obesity is increasing in most of the West and is more
common in people from lower socioeconomic classes. Medical means
of treatment should only be used with BMI <30 kg/m^2 and if the
patients show motivation by losing weight themselves. The South Asian
population has a different hip-to-waist ratio and may have risk of heart
disease despite normal BMI. Loss of weight in obese patients would
result in reduction of blood pressure.

4 Liver cirrhosis   Answers: B C

Publicans, boatmen, hotel managers, fishermen, chefs and journalists
are some of the groups most likely to die from liver cirrhosis. Ten years
ago doctors had a 300% greater than average risk of dying from
cirrhosis, but recently this figure has dropped hugely.

5 Retrospective studies   Answers: A C D

In retrospective studies great stress is placed on memory and past
history; bias is very common. They are cheaper to carry out and take a
shorter time to conduct.

6   Trials   **Answers: B C E**

The chi-squared test is a non-parametric test (data grouped by category) which is always carried out on absolute numbers, not proportions, means or percentages. The method is to construct a table using the data, then for each cell the expected number is calculated. The difference between the observed and expected is recorded, the result squared and divided by the expected number [(O–E)2/E]; the chi-squared statistic is the sum of all the values. The degree of freedom is (number of rows – 1) multiplied by (number of columns – 1). Potential confounding variables occur where there is some factor, other than the one you are testing, influencing the result.

7   Systematic reviews   **Answers: A B E**

Systematic reviews are the systematic, quantitative pooling of available randomised controlled trials (RCTs). The results of meta-analysis are usually presented graphically, with confidence intervals (typically 95%). They are not available for most medical interventions as RCTs are not available and commissioners are generally not in a position to use these in making decisions. Poor RCTs can produce wrong conclusions, as these will be compounded by pooled estimates of effect.

8   Studies   **Answers: C D**

The prevalence of a condition reflects the total number of cases in a population at a given time. Cohort studies may be used to study a defined group through time, eg a group of subjects exposed to a suspected cause of a disease at a particular time are then followed up to see whether they develop the disease.

The mode is the value which occurs most frequently, ie the maximum value on the frequency distribution curve. If a distribution is positively skewed with a long tail on the right side and more large values, the mode will be less than the mean. Similarly, if the distribution is negatively skewed (long tail on the left, more small values) the mode will be greater than the mean.

The standard error of the mean of a sample (SEM) is a measure of how accurately the true population mean has been estimated. It may be calculated by dividing the standard deviation of the sample by the square root of the sample size (SD/$\sqrt{n}$).

9   Standard deviation   Answers: B C D

The standard deviation is a measure of the scatter of observations about the mean. It is distorted by extreme values when compared to the range. Standard deviation is the square root of the variance. The standard error is a measure of the accuracy of the sample mean when compared with the unknown population mean. It is calculated by SD/($\sqrt{n}$), where n is the number in the sample. The chi-squared test is a non-parametric test and is carried out on absolute numbers, not proportions, means or percentages.

10 Statistics   Answers: B C D

$P = 0.01$ means that the results could have occurred by chance at 1 in a 100 observations, $P = 0.05$ occurs in 1 in 20 observations. The former is of greater statistical significance. Prevalence is the total number of cases (old and new) at a certain point in time. The incidence is the number of new cases occurring over a set period. In a chronic condition prevalence is much greater than incidence. In a short-lived condition prevalence can equal incidence. The mean is the average value, the mode the most frequently occurring value, and the median the value in the middle.

11 Study   Answers: A C E

The mean and standard deviation should completely define the normal distribution, with 95% of the sample data lying within an interval defined by the mean ± 2 standard deviations. The variance is the square of the standard deviation. In any study it is hoped that the sample mean will be equal to the population mean, but they are most unlikely to be exactly equal. Remember that the median is equal to the mean when the data are normally distributed.

12 Study   **Answers: C E**

Statistical significance does not imply clinical significance. In addition to assessing the clinical improvement produced by a therapy, account must also be taken of side-effects.

The chi-squared value is a calculated statistic used to compare proportions and has no immediate intuitive meaning unlike a P value or a mean. Any bias or confounding element (eg differences in the severity of disease between the two groups) may invalidate a trial.

13 Clinical trial of a new treatment   **Answers: B C D**

The null hypothesis is rejected if there is a significant difference between the groups. A type I error occurs when the null hypothesis is wrongly rejected (ie concluding that a significant difference exists when in reality it does not). A type II error occurs when the null hypothesis is accepted, when in reality a genuine difference exists between the two groups. The power of a trial is the probability of rejecting the null hypothesis when it is false, ie of concluding a difference or result of a given size is statistically significant. The power of a trial generally is increased when the number of participants is large and is decreased if the difference to be detected is small.

14 Correlation methods   **Answers: A C**

Correlation methods are used to examine whether there is a linear relationship between two continuous variables; the strength of the association is reflected in the value of r from -1 to $+1$. If the correlation is strong r has values of less than -0.5 or greater than $+0.5$. The statistical significance of a particular r is calculated separately. Even if a correlation is poor, it may still be statistically significant. Although two variables may be correlated, this does not allow a value for one variable to be calculated from a value of the second. Regression analysis and the derivation of a regression equation may be used to calculate the value of one (dependent) variable from a second (independent) variable. Mortality is not a continuous variable.

15 Mean   Answers: B C D

Normal distribution is not the only symmetrical distribution; many other symmetrical distributions exist. If the observations had been found to be positively skewed, their mode would have been less than the mean. The median time is equal to the 50th percentile. The variance of the observations would provide a measure of their spread about the mean. The standard error is a measure of the reliability of the mean value.

16 Referral rates   Answers: A B

Referral rate appears to be related to the individual doctor and not to the prescribing pattern or the size of the practice. Deprivation accounts for about one-third of the variation. GP experience in a particular field can actually increase the referral rate.

17 A GP's patients   Answers: B D E

(From Fry J. *General Practice – the Facts*)

Condition	Persons consulting per year per 2000
Acute bronchitis	116
Pneumonia	12
Acute myocardial infarction	8
(sudden death)	(4)
Acute stroke	6
Severe depression	10
(parasuicide)	(4)
Suicide	(1 in 4 years)
Acute abdominal conditions	6
All new cancers	8

18 The Oxcheck Study   **Answers: C D**

The Oxcheck study was a study of primary prevention in coronary heart disease. It looked at nurse-led risk factor intervention clinics in the General Practice setting. The clinics were expensive and the outcome measures showed disappointing results. However, the focus was usefully moved to secondary prevention.

SINGLE BEST ANSWER QUESTIONS

1   Clinical governance   **Answer: E**

Clinical governance demands that doctors take part in audit, examples of good practice are disseminated, leadership is developed within the team, evidence-based medicine is practised and that risk management is in place.

2   Clinical governance   **Answer: A**

Clinical governance involves efficiency, technical quality, risk management and patient satisfaction. It should help to show that self-regulation is appropriate for the profession.

3   Strokes   **Answer: A**

Strokes are very common and indeed are the commonest cause of disability. They are the second most common cause of death in the UK. Each episode of stroke has a 30% mortality, with a 10% recurrence rate in the first year. Twenty per cent are due to haemorrhage; 80% are due to infarction.

4   Study   **Answer: B**

A correlation coefficient is a measure of a linear relationship between two independently measured variables. It does not indicate a definite relationship. A value of 1.0 indicates a perfect positive relationship, –1.0 a negative one and zero the absence of a linear one. It is possible that in a 'U' shaped relationship, then, the correlation could be zero. The P value depends on the correlation found and the number studied.

5   Normal (Gaussian) distribution   **Answer: D**

In a normal distribution the mode is the most frequent observation, the median divides the distribution exactly into two halves; the mean, median and the mode are numerically the same. A Poisson distribution is discrete and relates to the number of events which happen in a fixed time interval. It can be used, for example, to compare death rates that can be regarded as happening by random event in a community.

6 Median   **Answer: C**

The median and mode are used in preference to the arithmetic mean when a set of values is from a population with a skewed distribution. In such situations values from the long tail of the skew distribution disproportionately affect the value of the arithmetic mean (average), which may be misleading.

7 Study   **Answer: C**

r is simply the correlation coefficient. There is a positive association between the two variables. A statistically significant correlation does not necessarily imply a causal relationship. The small value of P implies that the mathematical relationship present has been established as statistically significant, so more than sufficient infants were studied.

8 UK respiratory diseases   **Answer: A**

In the UK, respiratory diseases account for 20% of deaths and over 30% of sickness absence from work. Twenty-five per cent of medical admissions to hospital are due to respiratory diseases.

9 Wheelchair use   **Answer: A**

Over 20% of wheelchairs are provided for patients with arthritis.

10 Intermittent claudication   **Answer: B**

Many patients with intermittent claudication find that their symptoms remain static or even improve following presentation, particularly in the first two years. The clinical course is more benign in women than in men. Regular exercise improves blood flow in the long term and should be encouraged. Life expectancy is shorter than in unaffected individuals.

SUMMARY COMPLETION QUESTION

THEME: BACK PAIN

1	F	(randomised controlled trial)
2	C	(intervention)
3	I	(outcome)
4	D	(clinical)
5	A	(quantify)
6	J	(control)
7	B	(inconclusive)
8	K	(does not)

SUMMARY COMPLETION QUESTION

THEME: COX-2 INHIBITORS

1	H	(cohorts)
2	L	(non-gastrointestinal)
3	R	(cardiovascular)
4	K	(overall)
5	E	(stratify)
6	C	(gastroprotective agents)
7	I	(unadjusted)
8	P	(adjusted)
9	N	(higher)
10	T	(rofecoxib)
11	A	(NSAID)
12	B	(adverse)

INDEX

*Page numbers in normal text refer to the questions, page numbers in **bold** refer to the answers.*

abdomen, pain 55, 74, **251**, **265–6**
Access to Health Records Act (1990) 162, **316**
Access to Medical Reports Act (1988) 162, **316**
aciclovir 84, **273**
acne vulgaris 18, **228**
acromegaly 39, **244**
adenitis 74, **265–6**
adolescents
    contraception 129, **298**
    mental illness 195, **336**
    puberty 78, **269**
advance directives 170, **322**
agoraphobia 105, **284**
AIDS 163–4, **317**
Alanon 163–4, **317**
alcohol abuse 96, 101, 111, **279**, **281**, **289**
    voluntary organisations 163–4, **317**
    withdrawal 107, **286**
aldosterone 39, **244**
alkaline phosphatase 40, **244–5**
allergy
    alveolitis 139, **303**
    dermatitis 15, **226**
    rhinitis 27, **234**
alopecia areata 17, **228**
aluminium salts 83, **272**
Alzheimer's disease 111, **289**

anaemia 71, 141, **262**, **304**
angina pectoris 6, **221**
angioplasty 8, **222**
angus castus 81, **271**
ankylosing spondylitis 41–2, **245**
antibiotics 84–5, **273**
antidepressants 112, **290**
antidiuretic hormone 39, **244**
antiviral agents 84, **273**
    see also zanamivir
anxiety 98–9, 106, **280**, **284**
anxiolytics 85, 86, **274**, **275**
aorta 3, **219**
appendicitis 74, **265–6**
arm *see* upper limb
arthritis 41–2, 54, 79–80, **245**, **250**, **270**
ASH (Action on Smoking and Health) 163–4, **317**
aspirin 86, **274**
asthma 147, **308**
    adult 143, **305**
    British Thoracic Society guidelines 145, **307**
    childhood 143, 146, **305**, **308**
    diagnosis 139, 147, **303**, **308**
    treatment 145, **307**
atrial fibrillation (AF) 4, 7, 9–11, **220**, **222**, **223**
audiograms 28–9, **235**
audit
    clinical 187, 207–9, **332**, **344**
    economic 150–4, 184, **310**, **330**
average *see* mean

backache 114, 207–9, **291**, **344**
Balint, M, on consultation 189,
   333
basal cell carcinoma 19, **229**
bedwetting 77, **268**
Bell's palsy 109, **287**
benzodiazepines 85, 86, **274**, **275**
bereavement 106, 163–4, **284**,
   317
Berne, E, on consultation 161,
   189, **315**, **333**
bile duct 61, **255**
Biomedical consultation model
   161, **315**
bipolar disorder 98–9, **280**
bisphosphonates 38, **243**
bladder cancer 134, **301**
blindness *see* vision
blood pressure (BP)
   heart disease 192, **334–5**
   hypertension 7, 190, 193–4,
      222, **333**, **335**
   pulses 3, **219**
bone diseases, metabolic 40,
   244–5
borderline personality disorder
   98–9, **280**
bowel habits 56, 62, **251–2**, **255**
breast cancer 122, 132, **293**, **300**
breast-feeding 75, 88, 126, **267**,
   276, **296**
breathlessness 139–42, **303–4**
British Hypertension Society
   Guidelines 7, 193–4, **222**,
   335
bronchial carcinoma 147, **308**
bulimia nervosa 104, **283**
burnout 169, **321**
butterbur 81, **271**
Byrne, PS and Long, BEL, on con-

sultation 161, 189, **315**, **333**

café au lait patches 79–80, **270**
CAGE questionnaire 96, **279**
calcium
   bone diseases 40, **244–5**
   ECGs 4, **220**
cancer
   gynaecological 122, **293**
   infective agents 66, **259**
   see also specific sites
cannabis 85, 86, **274**, **275**
carbon monoxide poisoning 101,
   281
carcinoid syndrome 56, **251–2**
cardiovascular disease, clinical trials 191–2, 202, **334–5**, **341**
carpal tunnel syndrome 46, **248**
case – control studies
   analysis 115–18, **292**
   design 182, 185, **329**, **330**
case rates 164, 190, 201, **318**,
   333, **340**
cataracts 34, **240**
cerebellopontine angle tumours
   24, **232**
cerebrovascular accidents 110,
   203, **288**, **342**
cervix
   cancer 66, 122, 127, **259**,
      293, **296**
   erosion 123, **294**
chest infections 68–9, 146, 148–9,
   261, **307**, **309**
chest pains, treatment 150–4, **310**
chi-squared test 196, **337**
chilblains 22, **231**
children
   abdominal pain 74, **265–6**
   abuse 163–4, **317**

asthma 143, 146, **305**, **308**
breathlessness 142, **304**
consent 168, **320**
developmental milestones 73, 77, **265**, **268**
mental illness 195, **336**
SIDS 75, **267**
social class 195, **336**
urinary tract infections 132, **300**
Chlamydia 126, **296**
chloroquine 13, **224**
cholecystitis 55, **251**
chromosome disorders 65, 67, **259**, **260**
Down's syndrome 76, **267**, **268**
chronic fatigue syndrome 112, **290**
chronic obstructive pulmonary disease (COPD) 3, 144, 148–9, 155–8, **219**, **305**, **309**, **310**
ciprofloxacin 84, **273**
cirrhosis 196, **336**
climacteric *see* menopause
clinical governance 203, **342**
clinical trials *see* randomised clinical trials
clubbing 145, 149, **307**, **309**
cluster headaches 95, 97, **278**, **279–80**
coeliac disease 56, **251–2**
schizophrenia and 115–18, **292**
cohort studies
analysis 47–53, 119–21, 210–16, **249**, **292**, **344**
design 185, **330**
coital cephalgia 97, **279–80**

colon
cancer 60, 65, **254**, **259**
colitis 55, 56, **251–2**
diagnosis of disease 55–6, **251–2**
diverticular disease 55, 60, 62, **251**, **254**, **256**
colour blindness 65, **259**
Compassionate Friends 163–4, **317**
compensation neurosis 105, **283**
competency 166, **319**
complaints procedures 166, 175, **319**, **324**
complementary medicine 81, 88, **271**, **276**
confusion, acute 107, **285**
Conn's syndrome 39, **244**
consent 166, 168, **319**, **320**
advance directives 170, **322**
constipation 62, **255**
consultations
case rates 164, 190, 201, **318**, **333**, **340**
email 167, **319**
models 161, 189, **315**, **333**
continuing professional development (CPD) 166, 173, **319**, **324**
contraception
choice 124–5, 129, **295**, **298**
oral 81, 87, 127, 133, **271**, **275**, **297**, **300**, **301**
post-coital 127, **297**
prescribing habits 135–8, **302**
under–16s 129, **298**
contracts 167, 168, 172, 173, **319**, **320**, **323**, **324**
conversion disorders 98–9, **280**
corneal arcus 32, **238**

coronary heart disease
  angioplasty 8, **222**
  clinical trials 191–2, 202,
    334–5, 341
correlation coefficients 200, **339**
correlation studies 182, 204, 205,
    329, 342, 343
corticosteroids 38, 39, 145,
    243–4, 307
costs 184, **330**
coughing 146, **308**
counselling 163–4, **317**
COX–2 inhibitors 210–16, **344**
Crohn's disease 55, 59, **251, 253**
CRUSE 163–4, **317**
Cushing's syndrome 39, **244**
cystic fibrosis 65, **259**
cysts, sebaceous 72, **264**

Data Protection Act (1984) 162,
    316
deafness 27, 28–9, 164, **234, 235,**
    318
death
  bereavement counselling
    163–4, **317**
  certification 171, **322**
deep venous thrombosis (DVT) 6,
    221
delirium tremens 107, **286**
dementia 81, 98–9, 111, **271,**
    280, 289
depression
  postnatal 126, 129, 130, **296,**
    298
  risk factors 105, **283**
  symptoms 101, **281**
  treatment 81, 88, 112, **271,**
    276, 290
  see also suicide

dermatoses see rashes
descriptive studies
  analysis 155–62, **310–11**
  design 182, 185, **329, 330**
diabetes insipidus 39, **244**
diabetes mellitus
  BP control 192, **335**
  cognitive decline 51–3, **249**
  diagnosis 45, **247**
  eye pathology 34, 36–7, **240,**
    242
  management 47–50, **249**
  NSF standards 45, **247**
  pregnancy 44, **246**
  prevalence 190, **333**
diarrhoea 56, **251–2**
digoxin 89, **276**
disability 205, **343**
Disability Discrimination Act
    (1995) 162, **316**
disc lesions 95, **279**
distribution 197, 198, 201, 204,
    337, 338, 340, 342
diverticular disease 55, 60, 62,
    251, 254, 256
doctor – patient relationship 161,
    189, **315, 333**
Down's syndrome 76, **267, 268**
doxycycline 84, **273**
driving 168, **320**
drugs of abuse 85, 86, 163–4,
    274, 275, 317
duodenal ulcers 59, **254**
dyspepsia see indigestion

ear 22, 24, 25, **231, 232, 233,**
    234
  see also deafness
eating disorders 96, 104, **279, 283**
economic analysis 150–4, 184,

310, **330**
eczema 14, 15, 21, **225**, **230**
electrocardiograms (ECGs) 4,
9–11, **220**, **223**
embolism *see* thromboembolism
endometrial cancer 122, 133,
293, **301**
endometriosis 123, **294**
entropion 63, **257**
epidemiologic studies
analysis 47–53, 115–21,
135–8, 155–8, 210–16, **249**,
292, **302**, **310**, **344**
design 182, 185, 187, 196,
329, **330**, **332**, **336**
see also randomised clinical
trials; statistics
epilepsy 168–9, **320–1**
episcleritis 31, **237**
erythema multiforme 14, **225**
erythema nodosum 17, 19, 149,
228, **229**, **309**
erythrocytes 70, **262**
exercise 5, **221**
eye
lesions 32, 34, 63, **238**, **240**,
257
ocular fundus abnormalities
33, **239**
reddened 31, 33, 35, **237**,
239, **241**
retinal photos 36–7, **242**
see also vision

familial hypercholesterolaemia 65,
259
familial polyposis coli 65, **259**
fatigue 112, **290**
fibroids 123, **294**
fingers, clubbing 145, 149, **307**,
309

foreign body inhalation 142–3,
304
FP10 *see* prescriptions

gall bladder
cholecystitis 55, **251**
gallstones 58, **253**
ganglion 54, **250**
gastro-oesophageal reflux 23, 57,
231, **252**
gastroenteritis 58, **253**
General Medical Council 174,
324
giardiasis 56, **251–2**
Gingerbread 163–4, **317**
ginkgo 81, **271**
glandular fever 68, **261**
glaucoma 31, **237**
glibenclamide 89, **277**
glucose, hypoglycaemia 43, **246**
glue ear 24, 25, **233**
gonadotrophins 39, **244**
gout 41–2, 43, **246**
granuloma annulare 17, **227**
grief reaction 106, **284**
growth hormone 39, **244**
Gulf War illness 119–21, **292**

H2-receptor antagonists 57, 83,
252, **272**
haematuria 72, **264**
haemophilia 65, **259**
hand 54, **250**
hayfever 81, 145, **271**, **307**
headaches
diagnosis 95, 97, 101, **278**,
279–80, **281**
migraine 30, 100, 114, **236**,
281, **291**
hearing loss *see* deafness
heart block 4, 9–11, **220**, **223**

heartsink patients 169, **321**
Heberdens node 54, **250**
Helicobacter pylori 58, 66, **253**, **259**
Henoch-Schönlein purpura 74, **265**
hepatitis 67, **260**
hepatocellular carcinoma 66, **259**
herbal medicine 81, 88, **271**, **276**
hereditary diseases 65, **259**
Heron, J, on consultation 161, 189, **315**, **333**
herpes zoster *see* shingles
hip
    congenital dislocation 76, 78, **268**, **269**
    protectors 38, **243**
hoarseness 23, **231**
hormone replacement therapy (HRT) 38, **243**
hyperkalaemia 4, **220**
hypertension 7, 190, 193–4, **222**, **333**, **335**
hyperuricaemia 43, **246**
hypoglycaemia 43, **246**
hypomania 107, **286**
hysteria 107, **286**

ichthyosis 14, **225**
immune response 70, **262**
immunisation
    influenza 64, **258**
    pertussis 67, **260**
    pneumococcal 68, **261**
indigestion
    gastro-oesophageal reflux 23, 57, **231**, **252**
    treatment 57, 83, **252**, **272**
inflammatory bowel disease *see* Crohn's disease; ulcerative

colitis
influenza 64, 88, **258**, **276**
intermittent claudication 206, **343**
intussusception 74, **265**
iritis 31, 33, **237**, **239**
iron 68, **261**
irritable bowel syndrome 55–6, 61, 62, **251–2**, **255**, **256**

jaundice 61, **255**

Kaposi's sarcoma 66, **259**
Kayser – Fleischer rings 32, **238**
keratitis 31, **237**
kerato-acanthoma 22, **231**
kidney *see* renal failure

lansoprazole 82, **271–2**
learning portfolio 166, **319**
leg *see* lower limb
legal issues
    Acts of Parliament 162, **316**
    death certification 171, **322**
    Mental Health Act (1983) 94, 174, **278**, **324**
    seizures 168–9, **320–1**
    see also consent
leuconychia 13, **224**
lichen simplex 12, **224**
lipids
    familial hypercholestero-laemia 65, **259**
    heart disease 191–2, **334–5**
liver 61, 66, 67, 196, **255**, **259**, **260**, **336**
lofepramine 82, **271–2**
loperamide 82, **271–2**
loprazolam 82, **271–2**
loratadine 82, **271–2**
lorazepam 82, **271–2**

lower limb
  diagnosis of disease 79–80, **270**
  innervation 109, **287**
  reflexes 103, **282**
  ulcers 14, 20, **225**, **229**
lung
  cancer 139, 144, 147, 148–9, **303**, **305**, **308**, **309**
  chest infections 68–9, 146, **261**, **307**, **308**
  diagnosis of disease 139–42, 144, 148–9, **303–4**, **306**, **309**
  respiratory diseases in the UK 205, **343**
  see also asthma; COPD
lung function tests 148–9, **309**

macular disease
  age-related 30, 36–7, **236**, **242**
  diabetic 34, **240**
  scotoma 31, **237**
magnesium salts 83, **272**
mania see hypomania
Marie Curie Memorial Foundation 163–4, **317**
MAST questionnaire 96, **279**
mean 183, 198, 201, 204, **329**, **338**, **340**, **343**
measles 70, **262**
median 183, 204, **329**, **343**
medical certificates 165, **318**
medical records 162, 171, **316**, **322**
Mediterranean diet 5, **221**
menopause 123, 124–5, 129, **294**, **295**, **298**
menorrhagia 128, **297**
menstruation 78, 81, 123–4, **269**,

271, **294**
mental disorders see psychiatric disorders
Mental Health Act (1983) 94, 174, **278**, **324**
meta-analysis 182, 197, **329**, **337**
metoclopramide 83, **272**
metronidazole 84, **273**
migraine 114, **291**
  diagnosis 95, 97, 101, **278**, **279–80**, 281
  loss of vision 30, **236**
  treatment 100, **281**
MIND (National Association for Mental Health) 163–4, **317**
misoprostol 83, **272**
mode 183, 197, **329**, **337**
molluscum contagiosum 19, **229**
mononucleosis (glandular fever) 68, **261**
'morning-after' pill 127, **297**
mortality rates 188, 195, **332**, **336**
motor neurone disease 113, **291**
mouth
  cancer 25, **233**
  dry 26, **233**
MRCGP examinations
  advice x–xii
  description viii–ix
multiple sclerosis 108, 109, 113, **287**, **288**, **291**
muscles, MRC power scale 102, **282**
myocardial infarction (MI) 5, 8, 139–40, **221**, **222**, **303**
  ECGs 9–11, **223**
  post-MI medication 192, **334–5**
myopia 33, **239**

naevi 63, **257**
nails 13, 16, **224–5**, **227**
negative predictive value 181, **328**
Neighbour, R, on consultation
    189, **333**
neuraminidase inhibitors 64, **258**
neurofibromatosis 21, 79–80, **230**,
    270
nocturnal enuresis 77, **268**
nodular prurigo 12, **224**
non-steroidal anti-inflammatory
    drugs (NSAIDs) 87, 210–16,
    275, **344**
NSPCC (National Society for the
    Prevention of Cruelty to
    Children) 163–4, **317**
null hypothesis 200, **339**

obesity 179–80, 195, **327**, **336**
obsessive-compulsive disorder
    106, **285**
oesophagus see gastro-
    oesophageal reflux
omeprazole 83, **272**
optic nerve pathology 30, 31,
    36–7, **236**, **237**, **242**
oral cancer 25, **233**
oral contraceptive pill
    choice 124–5, **295**
    and other conditions 127,
    133, **297**, **300**, **301**
    and other drugs 81, 87, **271**,
    275
    prescribing habits 135–8, **302**
orlistat 179–80, **327**
osteoarthritis 54, 79–80, **250**, **270**
osteomalacia 40, **244**
osteoporosis 38, 40, **243**, **244**
otitis externa 24, 25, **232**, **233**
otitis media 24, **232**

ovary
    cancer 122, **293**
    PCOS 123, **294**
over-the-counter remedies 90–3,
    170, **311**, **321**
    complementary medicine 81,
    88, **271**, **276**
Oxcheck study 202, **341**

Paget's disease 40, **244–5**
pancreatitis 55, **251**
parathyroid hormone 40, **244–5**
Parkinson's disease 104, **283**
parotid cyst 63, **257**
patient records 162, 171, **316**,
    322
Pendleton, D, on consultation
    161, 189, **315**, **333**
penicillamine 13, **224**
peptic ulcers 59, **254**
pericarditis 9–11, **223**
personal development plans 166,
    173, **319**, **324**
personality disorders 98–9, 106,
    280, **285**
pertussis 67, **260**
pharynx, cancer 23, **231**
phototoxicity 21, **230**
pingueculae 32, **238**
pleural effusion 141, **304**
PMS (Personal Medical Services)
    172, **323**
pneumococcus 68–9, **261**
pneumothorax 141, **304**
polycystic ovarian syndrome
    (PCOS) 123, **294**
pompholyx 15, **226**
positive predictive value 181, 186,
    328, **331**
pre-eclampsia 128, **298**

predictive value 181, 186, **328**,
331
pregnancy
antenatal care 128, **297**
diabetes 44, **246**
flying 174, **324**
pre-eclampsia 128, **298**
skin conditions 16, **227**
see also puerperal psychosis
premenstrual syndrome 81, **271**
presbysacusis 28–9, **235**
prescriptions 170, 171, **322**
prevalence 186, **331**
prostate gland
benign prostatic hypertrophy
81, 130, **271**, **299**
cancer 131, 132, 134, **299**,
300, **301**
psoriasis
diagnosis 14, 15, 21, **225,**
226, 230
on the ear 22, **231**
exacerbation by drugs 17,
228
psoriatic arthritis 41–2, **245**
psychiatric disorders
in children 195, **336**
diagnosis 98–9, **280**
prevalence 190, **333**
see also specific disorders
pterygia 32, **238**
puberty 78, **269**
puerperal psychosis 126, 129,
130, **296**, **298**
pulmonary embolism 139, **303**
pulmonary fibrosis 141, 148–9,
304, **309**
pulses 3, **219**
pyoderma 79–80, **270**

qualitative studies 187, **332**
questionnaires 96, **279**

Ramsay Hunt syndrome 24, **232**
randomised clinical trials (RCTs)
analysis 150–4, 196, 199,
207–9, **310**, **337**, **339**, **344**
design 182, 185, 187, **329**,
330, **332**
heart disease 191–2, **334–5**
systematic review 197, **337**
see also epidemiologic studies; statistics
rashes 12, 14, 15, 21, **224**, **225**,
226, 230
red blood cells 70, **262**
referral rates 201, **340**
reflexes 103, **282**
refusal of treatment 166, 170,
319, **322**
Rehabilitation of Offenders Act
(1974) 162, **316**
Reiter's syndrome 41–2, **245**
RELATE 163–4, **317**
Relenza[R] *see* zanamivir
renal failure
and drugs 84–5, 86, **274**, **275**
prevalence 190, **333**
resonance, lung 144, **306**
respiratory diseases 146, 148–9,
205, **307**, **308**, **309**, **343**
see also specific diseases
retina 36–7, **242**
retinal vein 30, **236**
retinitis pigmentosa 31, **237**
revalidation 167, **320**
rheumatoid disease 54, 71, **250**,
263
rhinitis 27, **234**
rickets 40, **244**

rifampicin 84, **273**
ringworm 72, **264**
RNIB (Royal National Institute for the Blind) 163–4, **317**
rodent ulcers 22, **231**
rubella 41–2, **245**

saw palmetto 81, **271**
scabies 14, **225**
schizophrenia
    and coeliac disease 115–18, **292**
    diagnosis 98–9, **280**
    prevalence 164, **318**
    prognosis 108, **287**
    symptoms 106, **285**
SCOFF questionnaire 96, **279**
scotoma 31, **237**
screening tests 181, 186, **328**, **331**
seizures 168–9, **320–1**
self-harm *see* suicide
self-medication 90–3, **311**
    see also over-the-counter remedies
self-regulation 173, **323**
sensitivity 181, 186, 188, **328**, **331**, **332**
sensitivity analysis 188, **332**
septic arthritis 41–2, **245**
sexually transmitted diseases 126, **296**
shingles 72, 113, **264**, **290**
sickle cell anaemia 71, **262**
sickness certificates 165, **318**
sight *see* vision
Simmond's disease 39, **244**
skin
    drug reactions 16, **228**
    infections 72, **264**
    pregnancy 16, **227**
    rashes 12, 14, 15, 21, **224**, **225**, **226**, **230**
smoking 23, 143, 163–4, **231**, **305**, **317**
specificity 181, 186, **328**, **331**
spine
    backache 114, 207–9, **291**, **344**
    disc lesions 95, **279**
    nerve root lesions 103, **282**
squamous cell carcinoma 22, 66, **231**, **259**
St John's wort 81, 88, **271**, **276**
standard deviation 188, 198, **332**, **338**
standard error of the mean 188, **332**
standardised mortality rate 188, **332**
state benefits 164, **318**
statistics 181, 183, 186, 188, 196–201, 204–5, **328**, **329**, **331**, **332**, **337–40**, **342–3**
stings 21, **230**
stomach
    cancer 66, **259**
    gastroenteritis 58, **253**
    ulcers 59, **254**
    see also indigestion
Stott, CP and Davis, RH, on consultation 161, 189, **315**, **333**
stroke 110, 203, **288**, **342**
subconjunctival haemorrhage 31, 32, **237**, **238**
sudden infant death syndrome (SIDS) 75, **267**
suicide 104, 108, 112, **283**, **286**, **290**
surveys 187, **332**
swan neck deformity 54, **250**
systematic error 186, **331**

tachycardia 9–11, **223**
temporal arteritis 97, 101,
    279–80, **281**
tension headaches 95, 97, **278**,
    279–80
Terrence Higgins Trust 163–4, **317**
testis, torsion 74, 130, **265–6**, **299**
thrombocytopenic purpura 63,
    257
thromboembolism 5, 79–80, 139,
    221, **270**, **303**
thrombolysis 191, **334**
thyroid disease
    hyperthyroidism 56, **251–2**
    hypothyroidism 23, 45, **231**,
    247
    prevalence 190, **333**
tinea 13, **224–5**
toes, ischaemic 79–80, **270**
tongue, geographical 63, **257**
tophi, ear 22, **231**
training 172, **323**
    CPD 166, 173, **319**, **324**
tremor 104, **283**
tricyclic antidepressants 112, **290**
Turner's syndrome 67, **260**
Turning Point 163–4, **317**

ulcerative colitis 56, **251–2**
ulcers
    gastrointestinal 59, **254**
    leg 14, 20, **225**, **229**
unemployment 164, **318**
upper limb
    carpal tunnel syndrome 46,
    248
    hand pathology 54, **250**
    reflexes 103, **282**
uric acid, hyperuricaemia 43, **246**
urinary tract infections 132, **300**
uterus, cancer 122, 133, **293**, **301**

uveitis, anterior 35, **241**

vaccination *see* immunisation
veins
    DVT 6, **221**
    ulcers 14, 20, **225**, **229**
    varicose 21, 79–80, **229**, **270**
ventricles
    hypertrophy 4, **220**
    LVF 3, 142–3, **219**, **304**
    tachycardia 9–11, **223**
viruses, associated with cancer 66,
    259
vision
    blindness 30, 34, 163–4, 164,
    236, **240**, **317**, **318**
    colour blindness 65, **259**
    field defects 31, **237**
    myopia 33, **239**
    see also eye
vitamin deficiencies 71, **262**
voice, hoarseness 23, **231**
voluntary organisations 163–4,
    317

warfarin 87, 89, **275**, **277**
warts
    genital 66, **259**
    seborrhoeic 19, **229**
wheelchairs 205, **343**
whooping cough 67, **260**
Wolff – Parkinson – White syn-
    drome 4, **220**

yellow nail syndrome 13, **224–5**
yield 186, **331**

Z deformity 54, **250**
zanamivir 64, 84, 88, **258**, **273**,
    276